HANDBOOK FOR HERBAL HEALING

A CONCISE GUIDE TO HERBAL PRODUCTS

BY CHRISTOPHER HOBBS

BOTANICA PRESS, CAPITOLA, CA

AUTHOR'S DISCLAIMER

The following recommendations are for educational and health-increasing use only and not meant to be a prescription for any disease. If you are experiencing symptoms, I always recommend contacting a qualified natural health practitioner or physician for a diagnosis and total health program.

OUR COMMITMENT

We at Botanica Press are dedicated in our personal and professional lives to environmental awareness. We are strongly committed to recycling, and we gladly contribute a portion of our profits to the Nature Conservancy and other conservation groups. This book is printed on recycled paper with a minimum of 10% post-consumer waste, and the entire text is printed using soy-based ink.

♻ This book is printed on Simpson 60lb recycled paper.

OTHER BOOKS IN THE HERBS AND HEALTH SERIES
BY CHRISTOPHER HOBBS:

Echinacea! The Immune Herb

Ginkgo, Elixir of Youth

Foundations of Health

Milk Thistle: The Liver Herb

Vitex: The Women's Herb

Valerian, The Relaxing Herb

Usnea, The Herbal Antibiotic

Natural Liver Therapy

Medicinal Mushrooms

Copyright October, 1990
4th printing, July 1994

by Christopher Hobbs
Beth Baugh, Editor
Brooke Matteson, graphic design

Botanica Press • Box 742 • Capitola • CA • 95010

TABLE OF CONTENTS

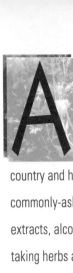

As a 4th generation herbalist with over 25 years of experience loving and using herbs personally in my daily life, I wrote this book as a practical guide to commercial herbal products available throughout the country and how to use them. It includes answers to the most commonly-asked questions about herbal formulas, single herb products, extracts, alcohol and glycerin (used to make extracts), herb quality, and taking herbs and herb products.

It also features in-depth information about formulas which I have put together over the last 10 years. These formulas are available in health-food stores, herb stores, and markets throughout the country.

THE BOOK IS DIVIDED INTO THREE PARTS:

1 An herbalist's practical view of the herbs and herb products available in natural food stores, herb shops, and from other suppliers, including:

- Herb quality--how to separate great, good, and inferior products.

- Women's herbs, herbs for children, and herbs that are safe during pregnancy.

- What about alcohol? Is it safe? Is it a good solvent? Is glycerin better?

- Why are organically-grown and "ecologically-harvested" herbs superior to "commercial herbs"?

- Herbal energetics and "Constitutional Herbalism"--understanding the concepts and applying them to make herbal medicine even more effective!

- Extracts--is "whole plant" better or "standardized extracts"? Are liquids more effective or "powdered extracts?"

- And more!

2 An herbal, describing the functions, energy, and uses of my formulas and a number of popular single herbs.

3 A complete prescriber, listing the formulas and herbs I've found to be effective for over 170 common ailments.

More specifically, you will also find answers in this book to some of the most commonly-asked questions about herbs and herbal products, such as:

What are the advantages and disadvantages of extracts and powdered herb products? Which ones are stronger?

How can I pick out the highest quality product for the best price?

Why is alcohol used in herb extracts? Is glycerin better? Are there alternatives?

What are the advantages of extracts made from fresh herbs-- or dried herbs?

Are organically-grown or wildcrafted herbs better?

What is herbal energetics? Constitutional herbalism?

What are the best herbs for children? Which herbs can be taken during pregnancy? What herbs should be avoided during pregnancy?

What are the differences in the way herbs are used in Ayurveda, Traditional Chinese Medicine, and Western herbalism?

AUTHOR'S INTRODUCTION

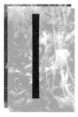f you ask herbalists what exactly they do, they will almost invariably answer, "Everything!" By this it is meant that they have been involved, at one time or another, with most aspects of the practice of herbalism. They have grown herbs, gone out into the woods and fields and harvested them, processed them, made a variety of herbal medicines such as tinctures, salves, and tea blends, learned the art of business and started an herbal company, and been a salesperson for their products, as well as an educator or herbal practitioner. Like many other members of the herbal family, I have done all of these things, but among my favorites is the art of formulation. Formulation of herbal products involves blending herbs together in formulas that can be taken daily to prevent disease and maintain health—as well as to treat a wide variety of ailments.

This book is about herbal formulas, many of which I have used in my own practice; I have also recommended them to other people for their personal use and to practitioners for their clinics. I have made some adjustments to the formulas over the years as new information has become available either from the scientific literature or from practitioner or patient feedback.

I have also included sections on herbal energetics, quality considerations, and information on the different types of commercial herbal formulas that are available.

Thirty-seven herbal formulas and twenty single herbs are discussed in depth, including sections on their energetics, actions of the individual ingredients, uses, and contraindications. At the end of the book, a Prescriber lists most of the common ailments one might encounter, along with the formulas and single herbs I have found to be effective for these complaints.

In this book, the reader will find a wealth of information on herbal medicine in a practical light—how to choose quality herbal products that meet specific individual needs for everyday health problems, as well as herbal tonic formulas that work well to support and strengthen body systems.

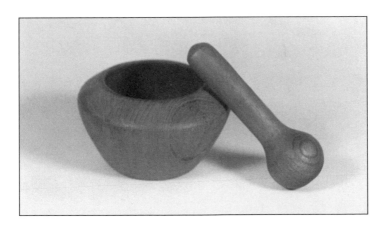

THE POPULARITY OF HERBAL MEDICINE

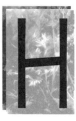erbal medicine is growing in popularity and becoming more integrated into the societies of western industrialized countries. This process is accelerating as the pendulum swings back from a place of "high tech" medicine where warm human contact and person-oriented medicine has taken a back seat to disease-oriented medicine, machine diagnosis, and industrial chemical treatments.

Today, many people realize that safe, gentle plant-based medicine offers practical self-treatment of mild everyday disorders, or even more severe ones as a first step before making that doctor's visit. Herbs generally place less stress on the body and its resources than synthetic drugs, and they are often less expensive. For example, for a mild to severe common cold, a prescription for penicillin, which may limit secondary bacterial infections, but won't do anything to bolster our own immune defenses, is $8, an antihistamine is about $30 (for a 2-week supply), and aspirin (name brand), $4.99 for 100 tablets. Taking the herbal alternative, a good echinacea/golden seal product should cost around $8, an antihistamine tea, about $5 a box, and willow bark tea about $3 (for a 1-week supply). Of course, the herbal treatment won't get rid of symptoms quite as fast, but it will work with the body to strengthen immune function, lower inflammation, and gently decongest. At the end of the cold, you will often feel better and stronger than before, instead of feeling like your body has been a battleground between powerful chemicals and the viruses.

For all these reasons, many people are trying the natural way first.

As recent studies show, up to 70% of the success of any remedy (and that includes drugs or herbs) is due to the placebo effect. So why not work with the body instead of trying to force it into submission? The primary goal in healing should be to let the body and its resources do their work unimpeded.

With moderate to serious pathology it is usually wise to seek the advice of a competent health practitioner or a physician trained in pathology. Most everyday complaints, aches, and pains will usually resolve within a few days or a week at most, and only require love, rest, and a simple self-treatment with herbs, diet, and other healthy practices. Self-care is a responsibility—we are in the driver's seat. By using our power, we feel good about ourselves and take our rightful place in helping to decide the outcome of our own evolutionary process as human beings.

As the year 2000 looms closer, several observations can be made that clearly show why herbal medicine may be of vital interest to many people on planet earth.

First, the resources of the earth are being used up. Oil and gas reserves are declining. The manufacture of synthetic pharmaceutical drugs uses up even more of these precious resources, as well as adding a further burden of pollution on already over-taxed ecosystems on our planet. The organic cultivation of herbs, on the other hand, is completely sustainable, creates good jobs, and adds beneficial substances, such as oxygen, to our world.

The population of the earth is constantly increasing, so there is more pressure on existing services and resources of all types. This includes medical services, such as patient care and medicines. This is due, at least in part, to our over-reliance on doctor-mediated treatments for mild, easily resolvable conditions, as mentioned above.

Second, it is well-known that the population in many parts of the industrial world is aging. Add to this the rapid environmental changes to which we have to adapt, such as increased radiation levels and a plethora of new chemicals in our water and food, and it is easy to understand why the demand for health care is rising, without an end in sight.

Third, although modern industrial medicine has many applications in the treatment of diseases arising through acute bacterial or other pathogenic influences (such as meningitis), as well as for accidents, its usefulness for most daily ailments and chronic diseases is severely limited. The manufacture and use of environmentally sound herbal health products as renewable resources make more sense for everyday situations.

Also, herbs can be considered "hightouch" medicine, rather than excessively "hightech." We need healing arts that are more person oriented.

WORLD HERBALISM:
3 MAJOR SYSTEMS OF HEALING

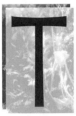here are three major systems of healing in the world.
In ancient India, the Rig Vedas spoke poetically about what
may have been the world's first organized medical system—
Ayurveda. This system is alive and well in today's India,
and its influence is just beginning to be felt in the U.S. and other western
countries. The second great system is Traditional Chinese Medicine, the
first written records of which are known to be from at least 3,500 years
ago. This complex system is an amazingly holistic one, in the sense that
the whole person—their constitution by birth, their living habits, and
environmental conditions throughout life—is carefully evaluated to
determine exact patterns of disharmony as well as exact treatment
protocols. Traditional Chinese Medicine, including its herbal remedies and
diagnostic system, and the manipulation of the physical body with needles
(acupuncture), is having a tremendous impact on health care in the U.S.
and will continue to grow at a remarkable rate in the next few years.
For example, a major insurance company recently instated coverage for
acupuncture treatments for coronary heart disease. This could not happen
unless the company was certain that the treatments would be valuable to
their members and save them money in the long run.

The third great system of healing is Traditional European
Medicine. This lineage traveled from the time of the first written records
of the Egyptians (about 2300 BC) through the Greeks, Romans, and

Persians to medieval Europe, the modern medical schools at Padua and Salerno, to the golden age of herbalism in the 1400s through the 1600s up to the modern day. This tradition is unbroken and is still a major influence in European countries such as Germany and France.

In Europe today, the European Community is crafting a single set of guidelines for the sale and use of herbal remedies—one that all the member countries will abide by. Thus the process of blending traditions is accelerating and is joined by a wealth of modern scientific testing that helps herbal medicine become accepted as a valid and important health-care partner by regulatory agencies (such as the Food and Drug Administration), political bodies (such as the U.S. Congress), and the medical establishment. The world healing system of the future will be a blend of ancient and modern—both art and science and heart and mind—because these seemingly opposite poles are not separate, but a part of the same knowledge.

Besides the three systems of healing mentioned above, there are many more systems that have been developed by various cultures over the centuries, such as Unani medicine and Native American earth-centered healing.

Interest in all three systems is growing rapidly. One of the main reasons for this is the frustration and dissatisfaction with modern industrial or "high-tech" medicine. People are instinctively seeking a more human approach, responding to ways of healing that seem to call us back to mother earth—seeking to be in harmony with the seasons and with our own natural rhythms. They are wanting a high-touch medicine.

In the U.S., and especially on the West Coast, we are at a crossroads. From the West we have the eastern healing systems coming in from the Orient and from India, and from the East, the traditional herbalism of Europe. We are very well situated and suited, by location and temperament, to take all of these rich influences and help facilitate a synthesis of them into a new world herbalism. As a diverse society with many peoples and cultures, we are also well-situated to synthesize these world influences.

A mass migration developed when many early Europeans came to this country in the 17th and 18th centuries, and they left many of their traditional customs behind, breaking the link with some of the traditional ways. Many of the herbs that they knew and depended on in Europe were unavailable in North America. This, plus the advent of modern, mechanistic medicine, may be one reason why our herbalism nearly died in the 1930s and 1940s. In the past 15 years with the advent of the worldwide "herbal renaissance", we have been able to take all the influences—from India, China, and Europe—and synthesize them, blending this art and knowledge with the earth-oriented influences from the Native American cultures, the African-American cultures, and others. This is the beginning of the new world herbalism.

This birth process is not complete, but what an exciting time!

CHOOSING HERBS THAT WORK— QUALITY FIRST!

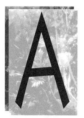n herbalist might spend years getting to know the qualities, energy, and properties of herbs, so she/he can effectively match the herbs or combination of herbs to the person and the situation. Obviously, some herbs are better for specific ailments than others. But equally important, and often overlooked at the store level, is the quality of the herbs that goes into a product. The identity, formulation, and quality of the herbs will have a strong influence on how well they work. Although a generalization, one would say that when choosing an herbal product for any ailment, whether mild or serious, keep four general guidelines in mind:

1 Make sure the company you choose to support has trained (preferably experienced) herbalists on staff who know and really care about selecting the herbs and making the herbal products you buy. Optimally, the personnel are dedicated to helping spread the "herbal word" through products and education.

2 Choose products that contain organically grown herbs. Make sure the sellers of the products know exactly where the herbs are coming from, so they can give personal assurances about the quality.

3 Vote with your dollars—support a company that you feel good about in all ways: environmentally, how they treat their employees, and if they love and care about their work.

4 For most cases, choose herbs that are in extract form, or buy a ready-made tea blend (or make a tea from garden-grown or fresh, high-quality herbs, if preferred), as they are more efficiently and rapidly assimilated and consequently often a better value.

HERBAL SOURCES: MANY WAYS OF TAKING HERBS

n India and other countries of the world, where herbs have been an integral part of health care for perhaps thousands of years, there are many different forms of herbal preparations. One sees myriad shapes and sizes of tablets and sugarcoated balls, pastes, extractions in honey or wine, and thousands more. In western countries, herbal products to be taken internally tend to fall into one of several categories.

MAJOR FORMULATIONS OF HERBAL PRODUCTS FOR INTERNAL USE

1 Bulk herbs—make a tea by simmering or steeping the herbs in water.

2 Herbs in tea bags, also prepared with water in tea form.

3 Powdered herbs (leaves, roots, etc.) placed into caplets or pressed into tablets.

4 Liquid extracts (also called tinctures or fluid extracts, depending on ratio of herb to solvent that was used to make them) are made by soaking the fresh or freshly-dried herbs in a solvent of grain alcohol and water. Powdered extracts come in caplets or tablets and are essentially liquid extracts with the water and alcohol removed.

Commercial herb products have a long venerable past and have much to recommend them. They have a few pitfalls as well, which can be avoided with awareness and care.

HERBAL POWDERS

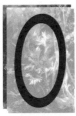

One of the most common dose forms found in herb stores and natural food markets is powdered herbs in caplets and tablets. Although whole and unprocessed (except for powdering) and reasonably priced as well, powdered herb products have several disadvantages. For golden seal and other roots that are fairly durable, powdered herb products are fine, where the ease of use and extra strength of extracts are not needed. For leaf and flower products and other sensitive herbs, powdering the herbs allows oxygen and moisture to quickly break down important active constituents. Also, many of the constituents are locked up inside the cell walls and are difficult for our digestive system to extract. For people who have weakened digestion or less than optimum assimilation, this dose form has less to recommend it than extracts. To summarize:

PROS AND CONS OF POWDERED HERB PRODUCTS

PROS

- Whole herb, minimal processing

- Low initial cost

CONS

* Reduced shelf life (perhaps to 1 year) because of large surface area of herb particles exposed to oxygen and moisture

* Absorption of active constituents is not as efficient as extracts because our digestive tract does not break down or digest the cellulose and lignin in the plant cell walls which lock up active constituents

EXTRACTS

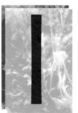

It is easy to define the word "extract." In the process of making an herbal extract, the active constituents or compounds are taken up into alcohol or water, which concentrates and preserves them and makes them easily absorbed by the body. Inactive constituents, such as starch, are left behind and not included. So an extract is a concentrated plant preparation containing a high concentration of active constituents and low concentrations of inactive ones.

ECOLOGICAL CONSIDERATIONS

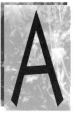 significant amount of fuel is consumed when shipping tons of herbal products across the country. Because extracts are more concentrated, they are more efficient to ship—less weight per unit of activity. It does use fuel to ship herbs from the grower or wildcrafter (or supplier) to the manufacturer of herbal extracts, but this cost is the same for both extract manufacturers and the manufacturers of non-extract herbal products.

EXTRACTS OFFER THE FOLLOWING ADDITIONAL ADVANTAGES OVER SIMPLE HERB POWDERS:

* Pre-digested, so are better absorbed, perhaps up to 40% more efficient. Poor digestive assimilation due to the effects of stress or stimulants is common—extracts are readily absorbed even when digestion is weakened. With extracts, the active ingredients are freed from the cells and cell walls that contain them, and they are rendered considerably more absorbable.

* Do not contain cellulose, lignin, and other indigestible cell wall components or starch.

* More quickly digested—liquids in 15 to 30 minutes, powdered extracts in 30 to 45 minutes, but powders may take up to an hour and a half or more.

* Absorption density is greater; because active ingredients are absorbed quickly, the noticeable or "experiential" effect is much greater than with simple powders.

* Time-honored method—Liquid and powdered herbal extracts have been made for thousands of years.

* The taste of the herb is concentrated and can play a role in the overall effectiveness, according to traditional medicine.

LIQUID EXTRACTS

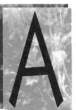 liquid extract is made by soaking the whole herb in a liquid that will release and concentrate its active ingredients. Water is the most familiar and commonly used liquid for this process, and one could say that a tea is an extract— the activity has been extracted from the herb, and the nonactive parts are discarded. This has several advantages. First, our digestive tracts will not have to expend energy in order to try and break down cellulose, lignin, and other plant structures where the active constituents are being held. Second, the active ingredients are concentrated and rendered soluble in our digestive juices, so they are quickly and efficiently absorbed. I estimate that many liquid and powdered extracts are probably over 95% absorbed, depending on the types of constituents involved.

Extracts are very commonly used in many parts of the world where herbal medicine is more evolved. In Europe, many extract forms are available and are undoubtedly more popular than bulk herbs. In China, and throughout the Orient, thousands of patent extracts are available and extremely popular.

One of the best aspects of liquid extracts is the ability to taste them. While the taste of herbs is unfamiliar to some people, or at times unpleasant, it is an important part of their activity. In Germany, it has been publicized, for instance, that scientific studies strongly suggest that the immune-activating properties of echinacea begin when the active ingredients come in contact with immune sensors in the mouth. When caplets and tablets are used, this activity may be missed. A bitter flavor is another good example. Through reflex action, when it is taken into the mouth, it can immediately have a beneficial effect on the digestive tract.

Liquid extracts (sometimes called tinctures) come in several forms. A tincture is usually made with a solvent, or menstruum, of grain alcohol and water. The proportions vary, depending on what the active constituents are for a given herb and whether they are more water soluble or alcohol soluble. For instance, Panax ginseng contains saponin glycosides which are fairly water soluble and thus can be extracted in a menstruum with a low percentage of alcohol, such as 45% alcohol and 55% distilled water. On the other hand, propolis, a bee product that is very resinous, is not soluble in water at all but must be extracted in 95% grain alcohol (ethyl alcohol) for the strongest product to be produced. Anything less in a propolis tincture will result in less active resins and flavonoids being held in the liquid—in other words, the value and strength of the tincture will be reduced.

To make an optimum quality tincture, just the right proportion of alcohol to water must be used. The alcohol has several excellent qualities and two others that are controversial—see the sidebar "Pros and Cons of Alcohol."

PROS AND CONS OF ALCOHOL

People often ask about the importance of alcohol in liquid extracts—does it have to be there, and are there any alternatives? First of all, it should be emphasized that alcohol is absolutely the best solvent, carrier, and preservative for the active constituents of most plants. An alcoholic tincture is usually stable (it will retain its potency) for up to 3 years or more (unlike 1 year for herbal powders in caplets); it is very quickly absorbed; and it is potent. The reason for the stability is twofold. First, the alcohol destroys enzymes the plant releases after harvest that will break down active constituents—enzymes that are still active in capsulated products, especially because they commonly absorb moisture while sitting on the shelf. Second, the liquid extract has only a small "head space"— the area above the line of liquid in the bottle where oxygen can work on breaking down active constituents. In powdered herb products, oxygen diffuses into the caplet and bathes the minute particles in the herb powder, providing a large surface area for oxygen to harm these delicate constituents.

It is also the safest broad-spectrum solvent available— much better than the methyl (wood) alcohol often used in Europe to create powdered extracts. Most high-quality herbal manufacturers use only pure corn alcohol, and every batch is individually tested using gas chromatography (GC) analysis for even minute traces of impurities (such as pesticide residues or heavy metals). This alcohol is proven to meet very stringent government standards for purity. Even "organic alcohol" should be tested batch to batch to insure no other contaminants are present.

The disadvantages of alcohol should not be a problem for most people, but they should be mentioned. A small percentage of people who take alcohol in some form will experience either a slight irritation, a mild allergic reaction, or addictive tendencies. However, I have known former alcoholics who had no trouble with liquid extracts—they did not activate a craving to return to drinking. I have not seen an allergic reaction occur in over 10 years of experience as long as the extract is diluted in water. Interestingly, recent statistics (1987) show that over 166 million people in the U.S. (64% of total population) consume alcoholic beverages, which is most of the adult population—in fact the average person actually drinks 2.5 gallons of pure ethanol each year!
(Special Report to the U.S. Congress on Alcohol and Health, Jan, 1990, Secretary of Health and Human Services, Rockville, MD).

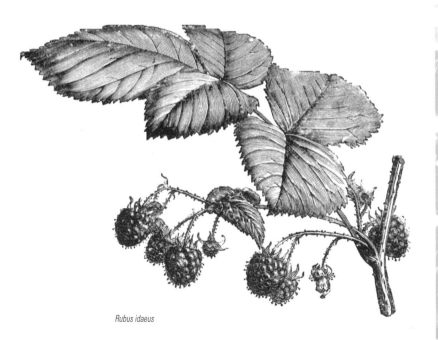

Rubus idaeus

WHAT ABOUT GLYCERIN?

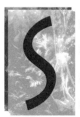

Some companies advertise "alcohol-free" extracts. These are made with the use of glycerin, which is similar to alcohol in its molecular structure. In weighing the benefits and liabilities of alcohol vs. glycerin, I have determined that alcohol is superior in several important ways. Like alcohol, glycerin has the potential to irritate the mucous membranes if taken without diluting it first in water or juice. Most importantly, glycerin is not as good a solvent as alcohol, and it will not carry the active constituents into the blood as well as alcohol. Also, commercial "glycerites," or glycerin-based extracts require more processing than alcohol-based tinctures, and thus important active ingredients might be lost. The only advantage of glycerin is it does not affect the nervous system, as alcohol can when used in sufficient quantity. However, when alcoholic extracts are properly diluted in a little water or juice, negligible effects on the mind or nervous system will be noted. Small amounts of alcoholic beverages, such as wines or beers, are thought to enhance health and digestion, and this view is being increasingly supported by scientific studies. Current evidence supports the idea that up to one drink a day can be beneficial to the cardiovascular system, acting as a digestive stimulant and general relaxant. More than this can increase the risk of cardiovascular disease, liver disease, and other degenerative diseases. As a comparison, a 12-ounce glass of beer contains, on average, 0.4-0.6 of an ounce of alcohol, while 6 dropperfuls of an average liquid herbal extract contain only 0.09 of an ounce.

In other words, one would consume about the same amount of alcohol when taking 2 dropperfuls of liquid extract 3 times daily for a week as in one beer!

The use of alcohol to make herbal extracts is of very ancient origin, being used in China, Japan, India, and numerous other countries.

To summarize:

ADVANTAGES OF ALCOHOL

* Excellent and efficient solvent

* Holds active constituents well

* Stimulates absorption of active ingredients (good digestive)

* Preserves the preparation for up to 3 years or more

POSSIBLE DISADVANTAGES OF ALCOHOL
(in the amounts used in liquid extracts when taken as recommended)

* Alcohol can be a mild allergen for some people

* Alcohol can be a slight irritant to mucous membranes when taken straight from the bottle—this is why many manufacturers recommend diluting in water, juice, or tea

Herbal extracts and preparations with alcohol are traditional, and herbal wines have been made for thousands of years. They were used by the Egyptians, Greeks, and Chinese; and in India, the tonic drink, Draksha, is a good example of an ancient preparation still made and widely sold today.

However, despite the many beneficial qualities of alcohol for making herbal preparations, some people will still prefer to avoid them. In these cases, the alcohol can be reduced by simmering the extract in a little water for 5-10 minutes, though the actual percentage of alcohol when the drops are placed in as little as 4 ounces of water is quite small, less than 0.1%! Make sure to store any liquid extracts that have the alcohol removed in the refrigerator, if the time they are used is longer than a day or two.

POWDERED EXTRACTS

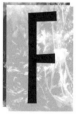 inally, there are other dose forms, such as teas, powders (already discussed), and also powdered extracts, which take the liquid extract a step further and contain no alcohol in the finished product. These kinds of extracts are in solid form, usually made by a two-step process. First, a liquid extract is made either with water or with an alcoholic/water menstruum. Then the liquid is dried, ideally under a vacuum, so as little heat as possible is used.

One common method is spray-drying, where the liquid is sprayed through a fine nozzle to create a mist inside a vacuum chamber. When a warm current of air is blown through the liquid, it is quickly dried, preserving delicate constituents. Because plants contain only very small amounts of "solids," or actual active compounds (remember that the initial extracting process removes the fiber, such as cellulose and starch), the liquid extract is actually sprayed and dried onto a "carrier" to standardize the finished weight of the extract and give it a little bulk to allow it to be encapsulated or tableted. The carrier might be a powder of the herb itself, pure cellulose, vegetable gums, calcium carbonate, or lactose. My personal preference is pure cellulose or vegetable gums, as they seem to be the most natural plant-based substances. The resulting powder can then be encapsulated or pressed into tablets. These kinds of extracts are ideal in several ways. When this liquid extract is dried, it is very much like the traditional method of making an herbal tea. In other words, the finished product is like a powdered tea. When fresh or freshly dried herbs are used, the resulting powder is an excellent representation of the original herb, minus the cellulose and other inactive constituents.

The potency of the finished product is not immediately evident. When a 1:4 powdered extract is listed on the bottle, that means that 4 parts of the herb were used to make 1 part of the extract. Or, in other words, 1 part of the extract represents 4 parts of the herb. This means that if there are 200 mg of a powdered extract in a tablet or caplet, the tablet really contains the equivalent of 800 mg of herb. Because of increased absorbability and efficiency of the powdered extract, it may equal as much as a gram and a half when compared to a powdered herb product. The powdered extract or the liquid extract is ideal for those with weak digestion and poor assimilation, or anyone looking for the benefits of herbs in a very concentrated form without having to deal with the bulk of dried powdered herbs, or the preparation time of making and storing teas.

STANDARDIZED EXTRACTS

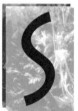tandardization means simply that the level of some constituent or constituent group (of compounds) is guaranteed to be a certain percentage of the total weight of the extract—within a narrow tolerance. For instance, one sees ginseng products that are standardized to 10% ginsenosides, milk thistle that is standardized to 80% silymarin, and ginkgo that is standardized to 24% ginkgo flavone glycosides. The manufacturer is certifying through laboratory testing, usually with high-performance liquid chromatography, that these products contain the stated amount of specified constituents.

Standardizing herbal products does have its benefits—it may provide more consistency in potency and help insure the correct plant is being sold. What about the drawbacks? First of all, we might say that there are two distinct ways in which herbal products are commonly standardized.

* An extract is made, using either water or grain alcohol, and then the levels of active constituents are simply detected and guaranteed to be above a certain level. The internal balance of the original plant is not significantly altered. I call this type of extract a "whole plant standardized extract."

* An herb extract is made with a variety of solvents, such as methyl alcohol, acetone, or hexane, and the active ingredients are isolated and removed from the parent herb. The finished product is made by concentrating and purifying these active constituents and blending them into a "carrier" (sometimes lactose or cellulose), or dried herb powder. In this way, the original balance of the herb is significantly altered, as one constituent is "pumped up" above its normal levels. I call this kind a "purified standardized extract."

Which kind is best? It depends on the use—they both have their place. My own recommendation is that purified standardized extracts be used by practitioners or educated herb consumers for pathology—in other words, symptoms are present. For instance, if someone has severe ringing in the ears, a purified ginkgo extract may be the best bet. These types of extracts are much more purified than whole plant extracts and are significantly different than the powders, teas, and even tinctures that have a long history of traditional use (sometimes thousands of years), so one cannot point to this use as an absolute test of safety. My feeling is that these extracts should be used for short periods as needed and then discontinued.

Whole plant standardized ("guaranteed natural levels") extracts are more useful for every day situations, for general tonic support, and for minor conditions, like the common cold or mild digestive problems.

The most compelling argument in favor of whole plant extracts is one that herbalists often point out—plants may have many active components, some of which are not identified yet and all of them work together to create a synergistic effect that can never be duplicated by a purified standardized extract. This view is also held by a number of German herbal researchers (i.e., Weiss). Over 500 compounds have been identified from some plants. During the process of isolating single active constituents, the synergy of all this plant's amazing diversity of compounds is lost. It is noteworthy that manufacturers have changed the constituent to which a number of common standardized herbal extracts, such as ginkgo, echinacea, and valerian, have been standardized over the last 5 years. This has come about because of constantly changing knowledge of the chemistry and pharmacology of these plants.

FURTHER QUALITY ISSUES:

FRESH VS. DRY

Extracts can be made from

* freshly harvested undried plants,

* freshly-dried plants or,

* dried plants, where the date they were picked is unknown (it could be 1 month or even several years!)

The second plants are picked, enzymes are released that start to break down active constituents. That is why plants should be dried as quickly as possible, without overheating them. This will immediately stop the enzymes. Grinding very delicate plants (like gotu kola) and macerating them in alcohol quickly after harvesting, while they are still green and fresh, will also preserve quality, because the alcohol will denature the enzymes.

It often takes years of research to determine what plants are best "tinctured" or extracted when fresh, which ones fresh-dried, and which ones will hold up well, so they can be extracted when dry. It is important to remember that while many plants are best extracted fresh, some are better dried, and some (like Chinese herbs) are not available fresh.

ORGANIC OR WILD?

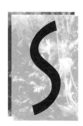 ome herbal product manufacturers will say that wild herbs are stronger than cultivated herbs, but this is not necessarily true; in fact, correctly grown organic herbs can offer better consistency. There is less environmental and genetic variation, and the growing conditions can be better controlled.

OUR WILD RESOURCES
ARE DWINDLING RAPIDLY

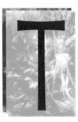he one overriding factor in the necessary shift away from wildcrafted herbs in the next 5 years is simply the preservation of our wild resources. We cannot continue to take the amount of herbs from the wild that we are now and have been for hundreds of years. For instance, for over 100 years, in excess of 50,000 pounds of the popular herb echinacea have been dug from its natural habitat—mostly in the prairie states and either processed in the United States, or shipped to Europe. Now, due to overharvesting in some areas and to widespread destruction of its natural range habitat, the wild resources of echinacea are rapidly dwindling. Golden seal is another example of an important medicinal plant that has been severely overharvested. This means that we cannot, with good faith, continue taking these plants from the wild. In fact, excellent quality certified organically-grown echinacea is available now, making it more important than ever for manufacturers to start using all organic echinacea in their products. In many parts of the world, such as Africa, a surprising number of the wild traditional herbs are almost extinct, and they are protected.

NO GUARANTEES WITH MOST "WILDCRAFTED HERBS"

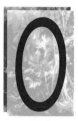ne more factor figures strongly in the importance of selecting organic herbs over wildcrafted (when available) —if a bottle of herbs says "wildcrafted" on it, there are no legal guarantees that the herbs in the bottle are good quality or free from pesticide and herbicide residues. A field of yellow dock can be bulldozed up next to an L.A. freeway and be called wildcrafted— there literally are no guarantees or legal guidelines. If in doubt about the origin of the herbs in the product you are using, I encourage you to ask the supplement buyer where you bought the product, or even call the company that makes it.

I don't want to sound too pessimistic about wildcrafted plants, though. A few distributors sell high-quality wildcrafted herbs that are very carefully harvested, dried, and stored. Some manufacturers of herbal products purchase their herbs directly from very ethical and caring wildcrafters who sustain their harvest by trimming the plants or replanting the seeds (as in wild American ginseng) whenever possible (Eco-Harvested). The only way to really be certain is by the reputation of the manufacturer — if a company really cares and is doing a good job in this and other ways to bring you a truly great quality product, the word does get around. And there is a further criterion—is the manufacturer a member of the American Herbal Products Association (AHPA)? The country's only herbal manufacturer's trade association is working diligently to help the industry increase its standards for quality and consistency. It has a Code of Ethics in place to assure that its members follow specific quality guidelines to insure the consumer of herbal products that they are buying the best available products.

KNOW WHERE EACH AND EVERY HERB COMES FROM

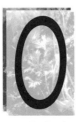f course, there are some fine products from wildcrafted or wild harvested herbs out there on the shelves. In some cases, such as the traditional herb osha, which grows wild in the Rocky mountains, there is no cultivation of the plant at all. So if one wants to experience the benefits of osha, it must be from wild sources. But some wildcrafters care about what they are picking— they won't pick next to roads and sources of pollution, and they won't overharvest a population—wildcrafting is an art. In other words, conscientious wildcrafters really care about the plants, as well as maintaining our precious resources, and not just profit.

The main question to ask the manufacturer of any herbal product is simply: "Do you know where each and every herb in that product comes from?" Do you know the grower or herb broker personally, or is the grower or picker reputable, and do you certify the origin of each herb? How is the herb picked and processed and what about the accuracy of its

identity? These say about as much about the effectiveness of an
herbal preparation as anything.

ORGANICALLY GROWN

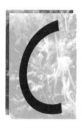ertified organic herbs must meet stringent regulations
concerning how they are grown and what kind of fertilizers
or chemicals were applied to the land in which they were
grown—sometimes for a period of years before any
cultivation takes place. A national law has been passed and will become
more enforceable in the future. Manufacturers will have very specific
guidelines about using the words "certified organic" on a product—
the major steps that go into making a finished product (especially growing
and processing) will have to be checked by a certifying agency. This will
make certified organic herbs more expensive and possibly more difficult
to obtain—this will be passed on to the consumer in the form of higher
prices on the finished products but will be well worthwhile, because
of the superiority of organic herbs over "commercial" herbs. Organic
farmers not only grow herbs, they start by growing superior quality soil.
In commercial farms, the soil is first sterilized with a fumigant or spray,
and the plants are grown with the aid of synthetic fertilizers. The soil
acts more as a medium to hold the plants in place. In the organic process,
the soil is considered a living thing—it is a whole ecosystem of insects,

worms, fungi, and bacteria. In this medium, the plants thrive and develop a powerful connection with the living mother earth. How can the medicine that is made from these herbs help but be superior?

To summarize, organically grown herbs offer these benefits over wild plants:

1 More consistency in quality, because of less variation in climate, genotype, soil types, nutrients, etc.

2 There are guarantees that no sprays are used. The plants are not picked next to the road or in polluted areas. It is possible to visit the grower to determine suitability of conditions.

3 Preserves wild resources, which are dwindling.

4 Supports the organic movement and provides work for people within a growing industry in tending the plants, weeding, propagating, etc.

5 More efficient energy use (gas, time, etc.), because the herbs are being cultivated in quantity in one place.

So ask for organic herbs and support products that contain them.

POSITIVE ASPECTS OF COMMERCIALLY AVAILABLE NATURAL MEDICINES

EXTRACT MAKING AND FORMULATION: A TIME-HONORED ART

Formulating and making herbal products is a time-honored art. Much thought and skill go into making a well-balanced and effective preparation. In the formulation process it is important to select just the right herbs so that the finished blend will activate or calm and nourish not only the system that is the main focus of the formula, but also work with other systems that may support the main system. In Traditional Chinese Medicine, for instance, if a person is experiencing fatigue and is under stress, it is likely that the adrenal system (the Kidney system in Chinese Medicine) needs support. But this system, known as the "mother", is thought to be nourished by the digestive system (the "Spleen" system in Chinese Medicine). Thus if any lasting results are to be found, the formula must not only support the adrenals, but the digestivepower as well; so a formula would, at the very least, contain eleuthero or schisandra (which supports the adrenals), as well as ginger and turmeric, to support the digestion. Of course this is a simplification; in actual practice, a number of other factors are taken into account. For instance, herbs might be added that counteract any tendency of the lead herbs to produce side effects in some people. Tonic herbs, such as rehmannia, may produce gas in some people, so ginger is added to counteract this. In my formulas, I often try to take into account nearly every system of the body. After all, our systems are all interconnected, and the health of one affects the health of the others.

In my understanding and practice of herbal medicine, I take what I find of value from traditional systems of herbalism—Traditional Chinese Medicine, Ayurveda, Native American herbalism, as well as European phytomedicine, and others. I am constantly in the process of integrating the ancient and modern understandings together into my own system, which I call "world herbalism." My formulations always reflect the expanding collective understanding of how the body works, how we as whole, unique individuals function, and how we interact with others and our environment. I strive to be a worthy conduit for the alive and growing energy of herbalism.

CONVENIENCE

In today's world, not everyone can be or wants to be an herbalist, wildcrafter, or herbal manufacturer. A finished product can save the buyer a lot of work. Sometimes, when we reach for that herbal product on the shelf of a store, it is hard to imagine the hours of work finding the herbs, cultivating and nurturing them, harvesting them, washing and trimming them, then drying, extracting, tabulating, formulating, labeling, educating, and so forth.

CONSISTENT POTENCY

It is the herbalist's and the manufacturer's job to insure that each batch of herbs meets certain standards. This requires experience, resources, and, of course, a significant investment of time.

CONSTITUTIONAL HERBALISM: A NEW, ANCIENT APPROACH

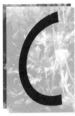onstitutional herbalism is a way of using herbs in a person-centered approach that considers the individual differences between people. For instance, instead of asking the question, "What is echinacea good for?", we ask, "Who is echinacea good for and under what circumstances?" Instead of giving echinacea to anyone who has the symptoms of an upper respiratory tract infection, we stop to consider other signs besides the obvious symptoms of runny nose, sneezing, coughing, and so forth. If the person is normally strong, does not have any long-term chronic immune weakness, and simply has an acute viral infection, then we can stimulate the immune system with echinacea to help mobilize the immune force and direct it towards the surface of the body where the viral attack is focused and achieve a good result. However, if the individual has had a series of colds or upper respiratory tract infections, or if the ailment has dragged on for several weeks or more without much improvement, then we have to consider the possibility of chronic immune weakness. In this case, an immune stimulant like echinacea would not be appropriate because it would be like trying to rouse a tired horse—the horse needs rest and care before it can go on.

Although it takes many years of study to fully understand the intricate concepts involved in Traditional Chinese Medicine or Ayurveda, there are several ideas that can help make herbal remedies more effective; for example, the idea that some people are deficient and need building up (use tonic herbs or formulas), and some are excess and need to have heat or energy removed or redirected to where it is needed (use specific or stimulant herbs or formulas). The first question becomes how to tell which situations require tonics and which need specifics.

TABLE 1

RECOGNIZING EXCESS AND DEFICIENT CONSTITUTIONS OR CONDITIONS

CONSTITUTION OR CONDITION	SIGNS AND SYMPTOMS	HERB OR FORMULA TYPE	HERBAL EXAMPLES
EXCESS	an individual has ample energy, does not feel chronically fatigued or run-down; is within normal body weight for their size and frame; tongue may have a yellow coating towards the middle or back, tongue body probably darker red; pulse on wrist is large, strong, bounding; often has genuine internal heat—generally avoids heat	specifics or stimulants that move and direct energy, usually cooling, draining energy	Golden seal, Oregon grape, Anti-Inflammatory Formula
ACUTE	a condition (such as an infection) that comes on suddenly in an otherwise healthy individual—no chronic fatigue or depression; tongue is red with yellow coating towards back; pulse is on the surface (it disappears when you press on it firmly), fast (more than 80 beats/minute)	specifics that cool and drain heat and mobilize the immune or nervous systems	Echinacea, Anti-Viral Formula, Colds/Infections Formula
STAGNANT	aches, pains, languor that dissipates during and after exercise—always better after movement, activity, or work; tongue has white coating, may be normal color or slightly red	specifics that warm, stimulate, and disperse	Ginger, Aphrodisiac Formula, Energy Formula
DEFICIENT	a person feels run-down, chronically fatigued (for more than several weeks); tongue may be livid red with no coating (a thin, white coating is normal) or pale (very light pink or lighter); pulse is thin, small, deep (have to press hard to feel it)—it feels weak or feeble; often has internal coldness or "false" heat—generally avoids or dislikes external coldness	tonic formulas	Astragalus, Reishi, Immune Deficiency Formula, Adrenal/Fatigue Formula

If a person has an acute condition and is also fatigued and run-down, then formulas or herbs can be taken together. Give a cool specific formula during the time there is an acute episode (like a cold or flu), and take fewer tonics during this time (tonics are warming and will often aggravate the heat of infection). After the fever, sores, headaches, infection, or other signs of heat are declining, then go back to the tonic formulas to build up the defenses and begin to taper off on the cooling specific formula. Many of my formulas detailed in this book contain both tonic and specific herbs. They are balanced for many types of situations and can be taken safely and effectively by people with different constitutions. Some of them are clearly specific or stimulating and some are clearly tonics. This information is given under the Actions section under each formula. See the section on Herbal Energetics below for more details about how to take Specifics and Tonics.

HERBAL ENERGETICS
THE FOUR PROPERTIES OF HERBS

Herbs are often classified into four categories, based on their energetic effect on the body:

PROPERTY	ACTION	EXCESS CAN CAUSE
Hot, warming	warms and activates functions	inflammation, rashes, headaches
Cold, cooling	cools, slows and retards functions	stagnation of energy, functions
Drying	counteracts dampness	loss of enzymatic function, heat to rise
Moistening	counteracts dryness	slowing of digestion, aggravation of stagnation

HERBAL SYSTEMS: SPECIFICS AND TONICS

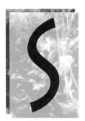**PECIFICS** are herbs or formulas that move the energy and blood and may change or stimulate a body process in some way. An example is echinacea, which stimulates the immune system. These herbs, which help focus one's vitality and energy into a particular function or process, are used for short periods of time for acute conditions (usually in cycles of 10 days on, 3 days off for up to 3 cycles) to do a specific job, such as protect us from a cold or flu. They are discontinued when they are not needed. If we need to take specifics for longer than these 3 cycles, we generally have a chronic condition and need to tonify our system on a deeper level. For instance, if we have chronic allergies, our immune system may be weak and unable to distinguish a non-harmful invader (such as pollen) from a harmful one, and it mounts an attack against it, producing symptoms such as red, itchy eyes and a runny nose. This is where tonic herbs come in.

TONICS are herbs and herbal formulas that nourish and support body processes and systems. Tonics work more slowly but on a deeper level than specifics. They should be taken for at least 2 months and preferably up to 6 months. Examples are reishi, shiitake, and astragalus, which tonify our defense system, or dong quai, which tonifies the blood. Here are a few points to remember about tonics:

* Tonics help to maintain tone throughout the body. "Tone" is a state of dynamic equilibrium, or balance, in the body.

* Herbal tonics are of two types: **1) Stimulant Tonics**, which are gentle, slow stimulants that invigorate and thus strengthen the body and its processes (think of the stimulation that muscles get during weight-training) and **2) Nutrient Tonics** that provide nutrients the body can utilize for its functions or in the repair process.

* Large quantities of tonics can be taken without the risk of over-stressing cells, tissues, or organs. The therapeutic and toxic doses for tonics are far apart.

* Tonics should be taken for at least three months, and up to one year.

This book covers formulas for body systems that act as specifics and tonics:

TABLE 2

SPECIFIC AND TONIC HERB FORMULAS FOR BODY SYSTEMS

SYSTEM	SPECIFICS	TONICS
BLOOD	Blood Purifier, Acne Formula, Heart Formula, Lymphatic Formula	Women's Bloodbuilder Formula, Menopause Formula
BRAIN AND NERVOUS SYSTEM	Relaxing Formula, Valerian, Headache Formula, Sleep Formula, Anti-Depression Formula	Ginkgo, Wild oats
CARDIOVASCULAR (heart and blood vessels)	Heart Formula, Brain and Memory Formula	Heart Formula
DIGESTIVE TRACT	Liver/Digestive Formula, Laxative Formula	Bitters/Digestion Formula, Milk Thistle
ENERGY/STRESS/ ADRENAL SYSTEM	Energy/Fatigue Formula	Adrenal/Stress Formula, Eleuthero, Gotu Kola, Reishi, 10 Ginseng Formula
IMMUNE SYSTEM	Echinacea/Golden seal, Golden seal Formula	Immune Deficiency Formula
INTEGUMENTARY (skin, hair, nails, joints)	Acne Formula, Anti-Inflammatory Formula	Lymphatic Formula
PATHOGENS, RETARD	Usnea, Anti-Viral Formula	
RESPIRATORY	Respiratory Formula	
SEXUAL HORMONE	Vitex, PMS/Hormonal Formula, Menopause Formula, Aphrodisiac Formula	PMS/Hormonal Formula
URINARY TRACT	Bladder/Kidney Formula	Bladder/Kidney Formula

** Specifics: take for 10 days on, 3 days off—up to 3 cycles; if longer treatment is needed, add a tonic formula, rest for 4-5 days, then take another course.

** Tonics: take daily for up to 9 months, or even years if needed; if desired, take a 3-day break every month, to evaluate progress; a minimum tonic program is 3 months.

Another way to match a formula or herb with a specific person and ailment is a more medical/pharmacological/scientific approach that talks about a state of imbalance or pathology in the body (such as inflammation).[†]

TABLE 3

WESTERN USES OF HERBAL FORMULAS

FORMULA	AILMENTS
BLOOD PURIFIER	cancer, skin ailments like boils, acne, headaches, other toxic conditions in the body
ANTI-INFLAMMATORY	arthritis, rheumatism, bursitis, colitis
IMMUNE STIMULANTS	colds, flu, acute infections (e.g. of the urinary tract, upper respiratory tract)
IMMUNE TONICS	AIDS/HIV, cancer, chronic fatigue syndrome, chronic bronchitis, cystitis or other chronic infections, candidiasis
ADRENAL SUPPORT	fatigue, depression, emotional swings, jet lag
ANTI-STRESS	overwork, protection against noise, pollution, heavy metals
RELAXING HERBS	sleeplessness, nervousness, anxiety
IMPROVE DIGESTION	gas, bloating, painful digestion, acne, foul breath, stools, inability to gain weight

The above chart may be useful for finding an herb or formula that will provide symptomatic relief for acute situations, or as supporting therapy for a more person-oriented energetic/constitutional approach. It does not particularly address the individual and their specific genetic make-up or the environmental influences that play a role in the condition.

†Please note that many chronic or serious conditions require the help of an experienced natural health practitioner or pathologist (such as an M.D.). Herbal programs should be considered as an addition to healthy life habits, such as a good diet, exercise, and a positive outlook.

HOW TO TAKE FORMULAS AND SINGLE HERBS

DOSES   When to take an herbal product and for how long

As a general rule, it is best to start an herbal treatment program, or begin ingesting herbs, with a small dose and work up to a full dose. In this way, it is possible to test for any individual reactions. We, as individuals, are the best judges of whether or not an herbal treatment is working. Specific action herbal remedies (such as golden seal) are taken for up to a month or so for a particular condition. They have a very specific effect and are taken only when needed. Tonic herbs, on the contrary, can be taken for long periods of time, even for years. Herbs are often taken in cycles. I prefer 10 days on, 3 days off, in repeating cycles. This way, the body has time to rest—there is also less likelihood that we will become accustomed to the remedy, and the effectiveness will be maximized.

The following chart gives the usual dose for whole herbs, teas, powdered herbs, liquid extracts, and powdered extracts.

DOSAGE CHART

DOSE FORM	DOSE
Fresh herbs (nibbling)	1 or two medium size leaves
Dry herbs (nibbling)	up to 1 gram
Teas	1 cup to 1 quart/day
Powdered herbs	2-4 caplets 2-3x/day
Liquid extracts	1-3 dropperfuls 2-3x/day
Powdered extracts	1-2 tablet 2-3x/day
Standardized extracts	1 tablet 2-3x/day
Highly purified standardized extracts	1 tablet 2-3x/day

The above chart is only an average, based on herbs that are fairly mild, with a long history of safe use. This dose is a good starting point, though even less is often better for the first few days, especially if one is not used to herbs or if a new herbal combination is being tried. Most herbs or herb formulas can be taken in amounts up to double the above, or even higher, when one is familiar with the activity or working with an herbalist or other knowledgeable practitioner.

CHILDREN'S DOSES

For children, use common sense. Take into account whether the child is robust or sensitive (or somewhere in between), the weight, the age, and how they generally react to herbal medicines in general, and adjust the dose accordingly. Always start with a low dose and work up to a therapeutic dose over a period of 3 days. Remember that children respond rapidly— the energy moves quickly in their bodies. Fevers come and go quickly, and their vital energy is usually good. Below is a chart of doses for children based on average weight and constitution. Give the drops in milk, juice, tea, or water. For a tonic herb formula dose, double the stimulant herb dose given here. The usual frequency is once in the morning and once in the evening—if a more severe ailment is present, consider adding a dose in the afternoon, but in this case, it may be wise to consult with an experienced health practitioner.

AGE	HERB ENERGETICS	DOSE
1 month	stimulant herbs	2-5 drops liquid extract
1-3 months	stimulant herbs	5-10 drops
3-6 months	stimulant herbs	10-15 drops
6 months-**1 YEAR**	stimulant herbs	15-25 drops
1-3 years	stimulant herbs	25-35 drops
3-5 years	stimulant herbs	35 drops-1 dropperful
5-10 years	stimulant herbs	1-1 1/2 dropperfuls
10-15 years	stimulant herbs	1 1/2 -2 dropperfuls
16 and above	adult dose	2-3 dropperfuls

** For children under 1 year-old, try to keep alcohol at a minimum—try a glycerin-based low-alcohol echinacea or relaxing formula.

HERBS AND PREGNANCY

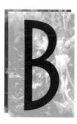ecause for the most part herbal medicine is gentle medicine, it is especially suited for use before, during, and after pregnancy. There are also a number of herbs that stimulate the uterus or are generally too stimulating to be safe during pregnancy—especially the first trimester, when hormonal levels are still fluctuating more than in the later stages.

Generally, avoid herbs that stimulate the uterus (oxytocic herbs such as golden seal), bowel irritants (my feeling is that is best to avoid laxatives during pregnancy), herbs which contain pyrrolizidine alkaloids (which may harm the liver of the fetus), stimulants (which pass the placenta into the fetus blood system and also are transferred to the child during breast-feeding[71]), blood-moving herbs (such as red clover or dong quai) during pregnancy and breast-feeding.

THE FOLLOWING HERBS ARE WELL-KNOWN FOR THEIR USE DURING PREGNANCY.

BLACK COHOSH   (take during last 2 weeks of pregnancy to stimulate uterus and prepare for the birthing process)

BLUE COHOSH   (take during last 2 weeks of pregnancy to stimulate uterus and prepare for the birthing process)

CHAMOMILE   (mild relaxer—useful for intestinal cramps)

ECHINACEA   (use low-moderate doses—up to 3 droppers/day maximum)

GINGER   (for morning sickness)

PEPPERMINT   (flavoring herb, useful for mild colds and flu)

RED RASPBERRY   (throughout pregnancy)

SQUAW VINE   (take during last 2 weeks of pregnancy to prepare for birthing process)

VITEX   (take during first 2-3 weeks of pregnancy— if you don't know you're pregnant until 2 weeks after conception, skip vitex use altogether; then continue use right after birth to promote milk flow)

* Caution: laxative herbs are generally contraindicated during pregnancy.

COMMON HERBS THAT ARE CONTROVERSIAL DURING PREGNANCY

(it is best to discuss the use of these with a qualified midwife or health practitioner):

BLACK COHOSH   some practitioners recommend its use for threatened abortion in the 1st and 2nd trimesters, but some say it should only be used in the last 2 weeks; probably best not to use it during pregnancy without the advice of an experienced health practitioner or midwife

BLUE COHOSH   see comments under Black Cohosh

CRAMP BARK   relaxes uterus

FALSE UNICORN   increases uterine tone but can be a gastrointestinal irritant in large doses

LICORICE   sweetening herb, anti-inflammatory but may affect hormone balance

PARSLEY ROOT   mild diuretic, urinary tract cleanser

RED CLOVER   moves the blood—may be useful in mild doses for blood purification

SQUAW VINE   tones uterus; (taken during last trimester)

COMMON HERBS THAT ARE CONTRAINDICATED DURING PREGNANCY

CAFFEINE containing herbs (Coffee, Chocolate, Kola nut, Guarana, Black tea)

CHAPARRAL may stress the liver

COLTSFOOT
(both Petasites spp. and Tussilago spp.) contains pyrrolizidine alkaloids and should be strictly avoided during pregnancy

COMFREY contains pyrrolizidine alkaloids

COTTON ROOT stimulates the uterus, used to induce abortion

DONG QUAI moves the blood

EPHEDRA contains the stimulant alkaloid, ephedrine (Ma Huang)

GOLDEN SEAL strong uterine stimulant; avoid altogether during pregnancy

OSHA moves the blood

PENNYROYAL the essential oil is an abortifacient and should be strictly avoided; the herb tea is much milder and is a good digestive herb

SHEPHERD'S PURSE stimulates the uterus, contains neurotransmitter precursors

TANSY stimulates the uterus, moves the blood

YARROW moves the blood, emmenagogue

HERBAL FORMULARY

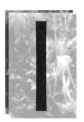In the following section, I present herbal formulas many of which I have used in practice since 1984. Most of them have been available to other practitioners and have been used in clinics throughout the U.S. They have proven to be safe, effective, and well-balanced for use by a wide range of people with a number of common health complaints. Over the years, I have made a few adjustments to the formulas as new research has become available and as my own understanding of traditional medicine has grown.

Some of the formulas are modeled after ones that have been available for hundreds of years or longer. Under each formula will be found the reasoning behind the use of the herbs that were chosen— why each one is in the formula and how they work together. Indications, or the ailments the formula will most likely benefit, are given, along with other helpful information about supporting the herbal treatment with other natural therapies. At the end of the section, the Herbal Prescriber will indicate which formulas are effective for various common health problems.

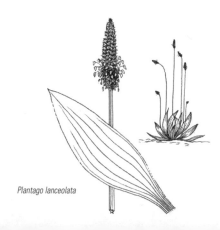

Plantago lanceolata

ACNE / SKIN FORMULA

INGREDIENTS: Oregon Grape root, Vitex fruit, Dandelion root,

Yellow Dock root, Burdock root, Carrot root

extract, Nettles herb, Red Clover flowers

Liquid form

Oregon Grape root, Carrot root, Vitex fruit,

Ginger rhizome, Dandelion root, Nettles

tops, Burdock root, Yellow dock root, Red clover

flowers, Food grown zinc, Food grown Vitamin C

Caplet form

USES: Acne (common acne, cystic acne, skin rashes).

This formula contains herbs that cool the liver and assist in the cleansing of the blood and lymph. Oregon grape is especially known for its beneficial effects on acne and other skin problems. Vitex is recommended for teenage acne in Europe—it may work by balancing the hormones, such as testosterone and estrogen. Carrot root extract contains large amounts of natural carotenoids, which have been shown to be beneficial for the skin. Nettles is a nutrient tonic for the skin, and red clover is a blood purifier.

ENERGY: Cooling, cleansing.

ACTIONS: Specific + tonic—cools, clears heat from
the liver and blood; activates elimination.

DOSE: 1-2 dropperfuls or 1-2 caplets 3 x daily.

CAUTIONS: Use caution during pregnancy.

PROGRAMS: For extra immune support, add Colds/Infections Formula; for extra liver support add Liver/Digestive Formula.

SUPPORTING THERAPY:

It is important to follow a cooling and mildly cleansing high-fiber diet. Refined sugars should be strictly avoided, especially in the form of baked goods that also contain oil. Stick to whole-grains, legumes (especially aduki and mung), lightly-steamed vegetables, fruits in season, and lots of water or cleansing tea (such as Polaritea: simmer 1 part each of fennel seed, fenugreek seed, flax seed, a half part of burdock root and dandelion root, and a quarter part of licorice root for 30 minutes. Take off the heat, add 1 part of peppermint, let the mixture steep for 10 minutes, strain and drink 2-3 cups warm a day.)

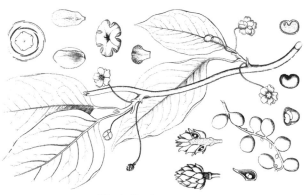

Shisandra chinensis

ADRENAL/FATIGUE FORMULA

INGREDIENTS: Eleuthero root, Ho-shou-wu root, Rehmannia root, White mulberry fruits, Ginger rhizome, Licorice rhizome   *Caplet form*

USES: Indications are for strengthening the adrenal system, supporting and releasing the vital energy of the body; in Traditional Chinese Medicine, a kidney yin tonic. It can be beneficial for periods of low energy and excessive stress.

This herbal combination has similar properties to Adrenal/Stress Formula but differs in being more for long-term use. It has a nourishing and supportive effect when the adrenals have been stressed for a period of time.

ENERGY: Slightly warm, tonic.

ACTIONS: Tonic—supports adrenals, nourishes blood, counteracts stress.

DOSE: 1-3 a day, morning and evening, depending on individual need.

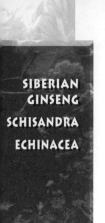

ADRENAL /STRESS FORMULA

INGREDIENTS: Siberian Ginseng root, Schisandra fruit,
Echinacea root, Wild Oats herb, Bladderwrack,
Gotu Kola   *Liquid form*

USES: Weakened adrenal function, jet lag, or
as a daily tonic to help adjust to normal
environmental changes and emotional stress.

Eleuthero ginseng and schisandra berries are two of the best-known and
studied adaptogens—natural herbal remedies that help us adapt to
stress.[76] A tremendous body of research involving thousands of actual
everyday use situations has documented these herbs' ability to restore
hormonal function, support the adrenal glands, regulate blood sugar,
increase the body's resistance to disease, and help counteract the
undesirable effects of stress. Specifically, they help us adapt to noise,
pollution, synthetic chemicals, radiation, or emotional distress—even
stresses such as moving or changing jobs.[77] The unpleasant effects of jet
lag seem to respond particularly well to this herbal combination. It even
tastes good, for the schisandra berries, known as wu wei zi, or 5-flavors
berries, contain all the 5 flavors (sweet, sour, salty, bitter, and acrid) and are
thus thought to be especially balancing to body systems.

ENERGY: Neutral.

ACTIONS: Tonic—supports adrenal function,
counteracts stress, supports immune function.

DOSE: One dropper a day minimum, up to 3/day
                   as needed.

CAUTIONS: None known.

PROGRAMS: With immune deficiency, add Immune Deficiency
                   Formula; with sleeping problems, add Sleep
                   Formula; with digestive problems, add
                   Digestion/Bitters Formula; with menstrual
                   problems, add PMS/Hormonal Formula or dong
                   quai; with depression, add Anti-Depression
                   Formula; with memory problems or mental
                   fatigue, add Brain and Memory Formula. For jet
                   lag, try taking a course of the Adrenal/Stress
                   Formula starting 5 days before the trip, until 5
                   days after.

SUPPORTING THERAPY:

                   When traveling, especially by airplane, it is
                   best to eat lightly. This leaves more energy
                   for the adaptation process—metabolic
                   adjustments take considerable amounts of
                   energy. Drink lots of pollutant-free (if possible)
                   water; distilled water is actually better than tap
                   water in most cases. Frequent stretching of the
                   body is beneficial in keeping the body flexible.
                   Hard physical exercise is one of the best
                   methods to counteract emotional stress.

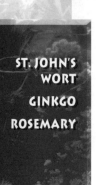
ANTI-DEPRESSION FORMULA

INGREDIENTS: St. John's Wort flower tops, Ginkgo leaf, Rosemary herb, Dandelion root, Black Sage herb, Licorice root, Cayenne fruit, Lavender oil, Rosemary oil   *Liquid form*

USES: Depression, tension, anxiety, restlessness.

Mild depression is a common ailment that many people are prone to at one time or other in their life. Stress, illness, hormonal cycles, and many other situations can increase the likelihood of one's experiencing "the blues." Medical doctors commonly prescribe various synthetic drugs, but these often place a further strain on the body, leading to even more severe health problems.

In Europe, herbal extracts are often used for mild, self-limiting conditions, where stronger synthetic drugs may do more harm than good. For mild depression, European doctors prescribe St. John's wort extract— time proven as a safe and effective medicinal herb. Modern tests show that it can counteract undesirable changes in brain chemistry that may lead to depression (MAO inhibitor).

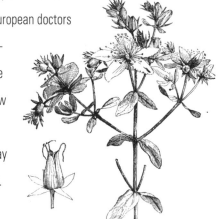

Hypericum perforatum

This formula contains St. John's wort and ginkgo, which also supports mental function by increasing blood flow to the brain and modulating neurotransmitters. Other traditional anti-depressive herbs include rosemary, sage, and lavender. Rosemary and lavender oils are included for their aromatherapy activity, also helping to lift one's mood immediately. Cayenne is a mild and safe metabolic stimulant, and dandelion helps keep the liver open and working smoothly (the liver can be an important contributor to one's mood; the old word "melancholy" comes from melanos = black and chole = bile.) It is the liver that creates bile. Licorice harmonizes the formula and adds sweetness.

ENERGY: Neutral to slightly warming.

ACTIONS: Specific + tonic—anti-inflammatory, sedative.

DOSE: 1 dropperful 3 or 4 times per day.

CAUTIONS: St. John's wort acts as a mild MAO inhibitor and should be avoided with synthetic pharmaceutical MAO inhibitors—it may sensitize the skin to light, so wear sunscreen and protective clothing during exposure.

PROGRAMS: For anxiety, add Relaxing Formula; for emotional swings, add Liver/Digestive Formula; for fatigue, add Adrenal/Fatigue Formula.

SUPPORTING THERAPY:
Walking, dancing, running, swimming, and deep breathing are all good for relieving tensions in the mind.

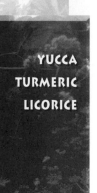

YUCCA
TURMERIC
LICORICE

ANTI-INFLAMMATORY FORMULA

INGREDIENTS: Yucca root, Turmeric rhizome, Licorice root, Chamomile flower, St. John's Wort flower, Black Cohosh root, Kava Kava root, Ginger rhizome, Barberry root, Chamomile oil *Liquid form*

USES: Arthritis, bursitis, athletic injuries, chronic bowel inflammation. Yucca, turmeric, and licorice are particularly noted for their anti-inflammatory activity. Licorice is included for its adrenal support, as adrenal weakness is a common factor in arthritis. St. John's wort counteracts pain and nerve damage. Black cohosh was considered by the Eclectic physicians to be anti-arthritic. Kava kava is a calming herb used for arthritis and rheumatism. Ginger has a warming, stimulating effect on the digestion, and barberry root is cooling to the liver and is recommended for arthritis.

ENERGY: Cool.

ACTIONS: Specific—relieves pathogenic heat.

DOSE: 1-3 dropperfuls 2-3 x daily.

CAUTIONS: With long-standing cases, try taking this formula with feverfew liquid extract, 1 x daily in the morning; with cold, deficient digestion, use with ginger tea or tincture.

PROGRAMS: For immune stimulating support, add Colds/ Infections Formula; for deficiency heat (weakened adrenals), add Immune Deficiency Formula; for stress relief, add Relaxing Formula or Adrenal/Fatigue Formula.

SUPPORTING THERAPY:

For arthritis and other heat conditions accompanied by fatigue and chronic weakness, make sure to eat a warm diet (i.e. fish or chicken 1-4 x weekly, mostly lightly cooked vegetables, and a variety of grains). Avoid sugar, fruits, and fruit juice. For arthritis or heat conditions associated with a diet rich in red meat, alcohol, and processed foods, eat mostly grains and a wide variety of raw fruits and vegetables. Strictly avoid red meat (at most 1 x weekly) and all refined sugar products and stimulants, such as coffee.

ANTI-VIRAL FORMULA

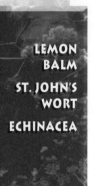

INGREDIENTS: Lemon Balm herb, St. John's Wort flower tops, Echinacea leaf, Licorice root, Wild Indigo root, Garlic cloves, Thuja leaf, Yerba Mansa root, Propolis bee resin. *Liquid form*

USES: Chronic and acute viral infections, such as chronic fatigue syndrome, AIDS, shingles, mononucleosis, and herpes.

Viral infections are among the most common and least treatable diseases known to the human race. Think of AIDS, colds, flu, and herpes. Viruses are thought now to play a secondary role in many other ailments, such as cancer.

St. John's wort was shown to inhibit replication of the AIDS virus by the National Institute of Health several years ago, and many doctors are prescribing the herbal extract for their AIDS patients—reports of some excellent results are filtering in.

Anemopsis californica

This formula includes melissa (lemon balm), which is widely used in Europe against herpes infections and is known to possess strong anti-viral activity because of its polyphenols.

64

A traditional combination of American herbs is also used in Europe against viral infections, especially colds and flu. It includes echinacea (which is known to increase the body's healthy cells production of the anti-viral substance interferon) and baptisia and thuja, both of which have good scientific backing for their anti-viral properties.

Isatis is a Chinese herb that has been proven to be powerfully anti-viral and is used in formulas given to AIDS patients in clinical trials in the U.S. Licorice is being tested as an anti-viral in AIDS patients in Japan, and garlic and propolis are two other well-researched herbs that inhibit viral growth and reproduction. Overall, this anti-viral formula will provide excellent inhibition and protection against a wide range of virus types.

ENERGY: Slightly cooling.

ACTIONS: Specific—slows viral replication, activates immune response, calming.

DOSE: 2 dropperfuls 3 x daily.

CAUTIONS: Avoid continued exposure to sunlight—St. John's wort may be photosensitizing to fair-skinned individuals; take with immune tonic herbs when there is long-term immune suppression.

PROGRAMS: For moderate to severe immune suppression, add Immune Deficiency Formula; for sleeping difficulties, add Sleep Formula.

SUPPORTING THERAPY:

A nourishing, warming diet is essential
for long-term immune suppression.

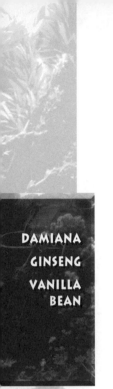

DAMIANA
GINSENG
VANILLA
BEAN

APHRODISIAC FORMULA FOR MEN

INGREDIENTS: Cacao seed, Muira Puama root, Damiana herb,
Chinese Ginseng root, Vanilla bean, Pine pollen,
Dendrobium stem, Passion Flower herb, Turmeric
rhizome, Kola Nut seed, Ginger rhizome,
Frankincense oil   *Liquid form*

USES: Impotence, lowered sex drive.

Cacao (chocolate) is one of the most renowned aphrodisiacs—it is
mildly euphoric and stimulating to the nervous system, with minimal
effects on the cardiovascular system. Chocolate and vanilla, along
with muira puama and damiana, are the most renowned aphrodisiacs
from Central and South America. Kola nut is a well-known stimulant
aphrodisiac from Africa. Chinese ginseng may stimulate the production
of testosterone and is considered an energy stimulant. Dendrobium is
used in China to support the sexual energy of the body. Passion flower
relaxes the body and mind, and ginger increases circulation and warmth
of the body, as does turmeric. Pine pollen contains natural testosterone

in small amounts, and frankincense is an aphrodisiac and blood-moving herb from North Africa.

ENERGY:	Warm, stimulating.
ACTIONS:	Specific + tonic—releases and directs vital energy to the sexual system.
DOSE:	2 dropperfuls as needed.
CAUTIONS:	Persons choosing celibacy should avoid using this formula.
PROGRAMS:	With digestive sluggishness, add Bitters/ Digestion Formula; with stress, Adrenal/Fatigue Formula; with anxiety, add Relaxing Formula.

SUPPORTING THERAPY:

The health of the whole body will support the sexual energy; a strong digestion, nervous system, and hormonal system will provide the basic foundation for a healthy sexuality; walking, deep breathing, hydrotherapy, and dancing can help free up vital energy and release tension.

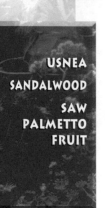

BLADDER / KIDNEY FORMULA (URINARY TRACT INFECTIONS)

INGREDIENTS: Saw Palmetto fruit, Marshmallow root, Sandalwood bark, Usnea herb, Horsetail herb, Licorice root *Liquid form*

USES: Cystitis (bladder infection), irritable bladder, inability to urinate freely, or other mild infections of the urinary tract. As a urinary system tonic and preventative, 1 dropperful/day.

This combination contains herbs (i.e., usnea and sandalwood) that act as urinary tract antiseptics to inhibit the growth of pathogenic bacteria in the bladder or other areas of the tract. One of the star herbs, usnea, has shown activity against some strep and staph organisms that is more powerful than penicillin.[1] Sandalwood is warming and antiseptic and was tremendously popular in the early 1900s in commercial cystitis and urinary infection formulas manufactured by Parke, Davis and Co. and others.[2] This herbal combination also includes soothing, demulcent herbs (i.e., marshmallow) to counteract inflammation and relax the ureter and urethra for easier urination, as well as general tonic herbs (i.e., saw palmetto),[3] to increase tonicity, elasticity, and nourishment of the tissues. Other herbs increase the flow of urine slightly, especially the release of waste products.

ENERGY: Cool.

ACTIONS: Specific—soothing to the mucous membranes of the urinary tract, antiseptic.

DOSE: One dropperful in warm water 2-3 X/day as needed.

CAUTIONS: Use for 10 days on, 3 days off in cycles as needed; if infection persists, consult with an experienced natural health practitioner.

PROGRAMS: For chronic conditions, add Immune Deficiency Formula; for extra immune stimulation, add Colds/Infections Formula.

SUPPORTING THERAPY:

Unsweetened pure cranberry juice is a good urinary tract acidifier (pathogenic bacteria generally do not favor a slightly acidic environment) and mild antiseptic.[4] Drink up to a quart of the liquid a day under most conditions. Beans (especially aduki) and rice, or other grains, should be the dietary focus. High-chlorophyl foods and superfoods can assist (spirulina, barley grass, chlorella, kale, beet greens, mustard greens, broccoli). Ample light exercise (especially walking), deep breathing, and rest are vital to successful treatment. Worry, fear, and cold are harmful to the kidneys and urinary tract—it is best to avoid them.

BLOOD PURIFIER FORMULA

INGREDIENTS: Dandelion root, Red Clover flower, Burdock root, Sarsaparilla rhizome and root, Echinacea root, Beet root *Liquid form*

USES: Acne, boils, carbuncles, dermatitis, cysts, tumors, foul breath, thick tongue coat, diarrhea, food poisoning, environmental sensitivities (with Immune Deficiency Formula); drug, alcohol, and cigarette withdrawal.

Herbalists often recommend blood purifiers for conditions like acne and other skin rashes, cancer, foul breath, and headaches due to toxicity. Dandelion and burdock gently cool and stimulate liver function; red clover is a classic blood purifier; and sarsaparilla increases the excretion of wastes from the urine (especially nitrogen-containing breakdown products of protein metabolism, such as ammonia). Echinacea stimulates immune activity and is considered a blood purifier and anti-inflammatory, and beet root strengthens the blood.

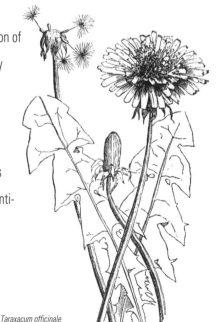

Taraxacum officinale

70

ENERGY: Neutral to slightly warm.

ACTIONS: Specific + slight tonic properties—moves the blood, enhances immune phagocytes to remove wastes from blood, increases enzyme production in the liver, increases detoxification mechanisms in the liver, moves and increase the bile flow, enhances the release of toxins from the bowels and urine.

DOSE: 2-4 dropperfuls 3 x daily.

CAUTIONS: People who bleed easily should use the formula sparingly.

PROGRAMS: For extra liver opening, add Liver/Digestive Formula; for immune stimulation, add Colds/Infections Formula; for removing heat from the liver, add Digestion/Bitters Formula; for constipation or excess heat-associated diarrhea or loose bowels, add Laxative Formula.

SUPPORTING THERAPY:

Add bowel cleansing, liver flushes, fasting, sauna therapy, hydrotherapy, vigorous exercise to the point of sweating (unless contraindicated because of weakness or deficiency).

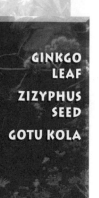

GINKGO
LEAF
ZIZYPHUS
SEED
GOTU KOLA

BRAIN & MEMORY FORMULA

INGREDIENTS: Ginkgo leaf, Zizyphus seed, Gotu Kola herb,
Wild Oats herb, Biota seed, Kola Nut seed,
Ginseng root, Shepherd's Purse, Nettle tops,
Sage Oil   *Liquid form*

Ginkgo leaf, Gotu Kola herb, Wild Oats spikelets,
Nettle tops, Kola Nut, Zizyphus seed, Shepherd's
Purse herb, Sage Oil   *Caplet form*

USES: Poor memory (especially enhances short-term
memory), muddled thinking, mental fatigue.

Ginkgo is a popular street tree in many parts of
the world because of its hardiness, longevity,
and beauty. Although used since
ancient times in China, modern
work has been performed to
isolate compounds which
boost memory,
increase brain
vitality, and sup-
port circulation to
the brain and other
vital areas of the body.
Gotu kola is a famous brain
and memory tonic from

Ginkgo biloba

Ancient India; wild oats is recommended by herbalists to support the nervous system; ginseng is a strengthening tonic; and biota seed and zyzyphus seed are recommended in Chinese Traditional Medicine to support and calm the nervous system. Shepherd's purse and nettle tops are sources of choline, which acts as a precursor for acetylcholine, an important neurotransmitter involved in memory and learning. A small amount of kola nut acts as a mild stimulant/tonic to the nervous system.

ENERGY: Neutral to warm.

ACTIONS: Tonic—moves the blood (improves blood flow to the brain, retina, and inner ear), protects vessel lining, improves neurotransmitter activity.

DOSE: 1-3 dropperfuls or 1-2 caplets as needed during the day.

CAUTIONS: Use cautiously in people with a history of stroke.

PROGRAMS: For general fatigue, add Adrenal/Stress Formula, Immune Deficiency Formula; for nervousness, add Relaxing Formula; for depression, add Anti-Depression Formula.

SUPPORTING THERAPY:

Like any faculty, memory gets better with use—you will find it improving daily when you exercise it regularly; take up a course of study, like a new language, and make it a daily part of your life; be moderate with fruit, fruit juices, and sugar-containing products, or stimulants.

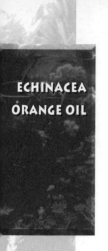

CHILDREN'S IMMUNE FORMULA

INGREDIENTS: Echinacea leaf, Echinacea root, Echinacea flower, Orange oil   *Liquid form*

USES: Colds and flu; respiratory, ear, urinary, and other infections.

Echinacea is the immune stimulating herb many parents trust to give to their children for colds, flu, and infections, but they sometimes have difficulty getting their children to take it because of the taste. This formula contains an excellent high-quality echinacea blend added to a flavorful, lightly-sweet base containing honey and vegetable glycerin.

ENERGY: In small amounts (less than 2 dropperfuls/day) spicy cool; larger amounts may activate the circulation and become spicy warm.

ACTIONS: Specific with slight tonic properties— activates anti-pathogenic vitality, focuses immune system resources at the surface to ward off viral and bacterial infections; slightly warming, dispersing to the blood.

DOSE: For all ages over 1 year, use 1/8 to 1/2 dropperful depending on body weight.

CAUTIONS: Long-term use in substantial amounts (over 2-3 dropperfuls/day) might lead to temporary immune suppression; contraindicated in AIDS/HIV without deep immune support; use cautiously in kids with autoimmune diseases.

PROGRAMS: For sleeping difficulties, add Children's Relaxing formula.

SUPPORTING THERAPY:

Gentle massage and abundant love.

CHILDREN'S RELAXING FORMULA

CHAMOMILE
CATNIP

INGREDIENTS: California Poppy plant, Catnip herb, Chamomile flower, Valerian rhizome, Lemon Balm herb, Tangerine oil
Liquid form

USES: Insomnia, nervousness, stomach cramps, hyperactivity.

Catnip, chamomile, and lemon balm provide a mild, safe, and effective combination of relaxing herbs, especially suited to children. California poppy was traditionally used by Native Americans to calm over-active children. It contains a number of non-narcotic alkaloids

Eschscholzia californica

that science has shown to be helpful for calming mild anxiety. Valerian is well-known to calm the central nervous system, which relaxes the body and mind, as well as supporting the sleep process at night, helping to provide a refreshing night's sleep. Tangerine oil adds flavor and is a mild relaxant.

ENERGY: Slightly warm.

ACTIONS: Specific with slight tonic properties— relaxes and calms; promotes sleep.

DOSE: 1-3 dropperfuls, depending on age and need.

CAUTIONS: Not for children under 1 year of age.

SUPPORTING THERAPY:

Love and attention; a soothing touch and gentle massage do wonders for a tense or overactive child.

COLDS, INFECTIONS, FLU FORMULA

ECHINACEA
GOLDEN
SEAL
YERBA
MANSA

INGREDIENTS: Echinacea root, Golden seal rhizome and root, Osha root, Yerba Mansa root, California Spikenard rhizome, Wild Ginger rhizome
Liquid form

USES: For the prevention and elimination of colds, flu, sore throat, and chronic infections, such as candidiasis and Epstein-Barr syndrome, in the acute phase.

This formula is a powerful "protective shield" combination, containing the most revered defense herbs from Native American Indian tribes around the United States. Echinacea was the favorite protective herb of the plains states,[5] osha of the Rocky Mountains,[6] yerba mansa[7] in the Southwest and Northern Mexico, California spikenard in California and southern Oregon,[8] and golden seal of the Eastern Indian nations.[9] Colds/Infections Formula stimulates blood purification by increased immune activity. It stimulates the surface immune system, helping the body to fight infections, colds, and flu. It is best taken in substantial amounts as needed before illness or especially in the early stages, though during illness it will also be effective. Take for 10 days to 2 weeks for best results, then rest for several days before taking again. For long-term exercise of the "protective shield," take 10-15 drops combined with Immune Deficiency Formula. Echinacea is a "surface immune herb," increasing the activity of the macrophages (the garbage-disposal system of the body).[10] Golden seal is commonly recommended by herbalists to help strengthen the mucous membranes and remove excess mucus;[11] it is also anti-bacterial and enhances digestion (being bitter).[12] Osha is known as a strong anti-bacterial herb and is warming to the mucous membranes and digestion. Yerba mansa is also a powerful anti-bacterial and immune adjuvant, according to traditional use, and California spikenard is a traditional cold and flu herb of the California Indians. This is a strong-tasting blend of powerfully-acting herbs, so people usually prefer to take it in water or tea to modify the taste.

ENERGY: Spicy warm, stimulating.

ACTIONS: Specific—stimulates immune function,
            especially the surface-acting protective
            functions; anti-viral.

DOSE: One to two dropperfuls in warm water as
            needed, up to 5/day.

CAUTIONS: Continued use in large amounts (over 2-3
            droppers/day) beyond 3 weeks may lead
            to immune suppression, especially in people
            with deficiency conditions.

SUPPORTING THERAPY:

Warm, eliminative, or sweat-promoting teas
are helpful. The classic combination is 1 part
each of yarrow, elder flowers, and peppermint.
Make an infusion and drink 1 or 2 cups during
the morning and evening. A traditional sweat-
lodge for purification (or more modern sauna)
helps to balance the energy of the body and
increase elimination. Eat lightly and especially
do not overeat—this uses a tremendous amount
of energy the body needs for elimination and
balancing. Eat lots of fresh vegetables
lightly-steamed, or in the warmer months,
raw vegetables and some raw fruits, such

as apples and grapefruit. Make freshly-squeezed lemonade by adding the juice of 1 lemon (organic, when available) to 1 quart of water and adding 1 teaspoon of honey. Drink the entire quart during the course of the day. For coughs, sage and lemon tea with honey is wonderful.

DIGESTION / BITTERS FORMULA

GINGER
ARTICHOKE
ORANGE
PEEL

INGREDIENTS: Orange peel, Artichoke leaf, Angelica root, Tangerine peel, Hops strobiles, Licorice root, Cinnamon bark, Cardamon seed, Gentian root, California Coast Sage herb, Tangerine oil, Ginger oil   *Liquid form*

USES: Poor digestion, bloating, lack of appetite, anemia, weakness due to chronic illness, constipation, gas.

In most cultures of the world, rich flavors such as bitter, sour, and aromatic are known to help promote digestion. An amazing variety of traditional herbal-based preparations that offer these beneficial tastes can be found in restaurants and markets all over the world. In Germany, where the importance of good assimilation of nutrients and prompt elimination of wastes is well-known, over 40 million doses of bitters are consumed each day. Bitter and aromatic-tasting herbal formulas are called "bitters." A variety of bitters can even be found in American liquor stores—various tonic waters also contain extracts of bitter herbs. Because our digestion is truly the foundation of health, bitters have been traditionally recommended by herbalists for a wide variety of imbalances.

Gentiana sp.

The Digestion/Bitters Formula contains bitter and aromatic herbs in an organic base to provide a bitter formula with the broadest range of beneficial flavors. Such bitter tonic and bile-activating herbs as gentian, artichoke, etc. are specially blended in a sweet organic base to make them as delicious as they are effective.

ENERGY: Warming.

ACTIONS: Stimulating tonic—activates gastric secretion of hydrochloric acid and other digestive enzymes, such as bile. Increases strength and tone of autonomic nervous system which energizes the digestive organs. Activates the immune system.

DOSE: 1 dropperful 1/2 hour before meals (this formula is most effective when taken over a few months time period).

CAUTIONS: Avoid bitters formulas with excess stomach heat (with symptoms of styes, gastritis, or ulcers of the esophagus, stomach, or duodenum).

PROGRAMS: With poor fat digestion, gas, and painful digestion, add Liver Cleansing Formula.

SUPPORTING THERAPY: When digestive difficulties occur, it is good to emphasize small meals of whole grain porridges (corn, oats, rice, and barley), which are easy to digest. Avoiding drinking liquids (especially cold ones) at meal time can create better digestion.

ECHINACEA BLEND

ECHINACEA
ROOT

ECHINACEA
FLOWER

ECHINACEA
LEAF

INGREDIENTS: Echinacea root, Echinacea flower, Echinacea leaf   *Liquid form*

Echinacea root, Echinacea flowering tops
Caplet form

USES: Colds and flu; respiratory, urinary, and other infections.

The best-known herb for colds, flu, and infections and an important "surface" immune activator. Used for the onset of all viral infections of the mucous membranes—sinus, nasal, throat, lungs, bronchi; also for lymphatic swelling. Speeds regeneration of new tissue for faster wound-healing. Shows anti-viral properties, increases the activity and effectiveness of the phagocytes (cell-eaters), especially the macrophages (big-eaters), to clear out old cells, pathogens, or toxins from the blood (what used to be called a 'blood-purifier').[26] Because scientific testing has shown both *E. purpurea* and *E. angustifolia* to be excellent in their own right, a preparation containing both species is to be desired.

ENERGY: In small amounts (less than 2 dropperfuls/day), spicy cool; larger amounts may activate the circulation and become spicy warm.

ACTIONS: Specific + slight tonic properties—activates anti-pathogenic vitality, focuses immune system resources at the surface to ward off viral and bacterial infections; slightly warming, dispersing to the blood.

DOSE: Varies with severity of the condition. For complete practical information on echinacea and its uses, see the book *Echinacea! The Immune Herb.*[27]

82

CAUTIONS: With moderate to severe deficiency, do not use without tonic herb support (such as Immune Deficiency Formula); otherwise it could depress immune function or T-helper cell levels when taken in substantial amounts (more than 1 dropperful/day) for over 2-3 weeks, especially with pre-existing immune deficiency. According to official German guidelines, it is contraindicated for autoimmune disease (such as lupus) and HIV infection.

CONDITION	FORMULAS TO ADD	ADDITIONAL COMMENTS
AIDS/HIV	Immune Deficiency Formula, Anti-Viral Formula (contains small amount of Echinacea to "energize" surface immunity)	take Echinacea mainly during acute opportunistic infections, colds, flu; otherwise in small doses (less than 40 drops/day) with tonic prgram
CANCER	Immune Deficiency Formula, Blood Purifier	best to work with a qualified health practitioner and physician
GUM INFECTIONS	Mouth-Care Formula careful oral hygiene is essential	careful oral hygiene is essential
CANDIDA	Immune Deficiency Formula, Echinacea formula	add a good probiotics formula (acidophilus, etc.)
CHRONIC FATIGUE	Adrenal/Fatigue Formula	plenty of rest and a mostly cooked-foods diet with abstinence from sugar and stimulants are recommended

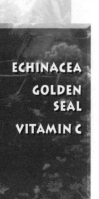

ECHINACEA / VITAMIN C
HERBAL COMBINATION

INGREDIENTS: Echinacea concentrate, Golden Seal

concentrate, Food-bound Vitamin C

Caplet form

USES: Excellent support for colds, flu, and infections,

especially when there is irritation or inflam-

mation in the mucous membranes (such as

in the sinus cavity, urinary tract, or colon).

Echinacea purpurea

Energetically, the formula is not

at all irritating; rather it is cool in

nature. This formula combines a full-

spectrum, all-organic Echinacea concentrate

(*E. angustifolia* and *E. purpurea*, double

extraction) with a Golden seal concentrate,

retaining the important essential oil

and food-bound vitamin C.

DOSE: 1-2 caplets 2-3x/day as needed.

84

ENERGY / FATIGUE FORMULA

INGREDIENTS: Damiana herb, Wild Oats herb in seed,
Cacao seed, Sarsaparilla rhizome, Korean
Ginseng root, Ginger rhizome, Rosemary oil
Liquid form

USES: Before sports activities, in the morning or any
time, to enhance the natural energy release
of the body.

Avena fatua

This formula contains herbs that warm
and stimulate glandular function,
digestion, blood, and nerves. The
rationale is to stimulate the release and
utilization of energy by the body but not
deplete its reserves, as do strong stimulants,
such as coffee or ma huang extract. The formula in
liquid form is readily absorbed and goes to work within a
few minutes. Rosemary oil contains natural camphor,[28]
which has been used for centuries to stimulate nerve
function,[29],[30] and in the ancient Indian system of medicine
(Ayurveda), to strengthen nerves.[31] Other supporting herbs
include *Avena fatua* (wild oats), often recommended by herbalists
for its nerve-strengthening properties,[32] ginger to warm the digestion and
activate the circulation,[33] which increases the assimilation and utilization
of the other herbs, and *Theobroma* (chocolate bean extract), containing

natural theobromine (0.5 to 2.5%),[34] a mild stimulant alkaloid which shows almost no stimulation of the central nervous system, but does provide a mild "experiential" energy lift[35],[36] (the caffeine in coffee, tea, and cola drinks is a powerful central nervous system stimulant). *Theobroma* also contains very small amounts of caffeine (normally less than 1%),[37] but when recommended doses of Energy/Fatigue Formula are taken, any effect of the caffeine is close to negligible. In addition, any detrimental effects of the alkaloid are counteracted by ginger and the other nerve tonic herbs.

ENERGY: Spicy warm; specific.

ACTIONS: Specific + tonic—warms and stimulates glandular function, digestion, blood, and nerves; stimulates the release and utilization of energy by the body.

DOSE: One dropperful in warm water or one caplet as needed.

CAUTIONS: Use sparingly or not at all for moderate to severe deficiency (weakness of the adrenals coupled with fatigue) conditions with signs of pathological heat (headaches, mouth sores, chronic, low-grade bowel or urinary tract infections, etc.).

PROGRAMS:

CONDITION	FORMULAS TO ADD	ADDITIONAL COMMENTS
LOW SEX DRIVE	Aphrodisiac Formula	use tonic formulas to build up general strength, Vitex for hormonal balance
DEPRESSION	Anti-Depression Formula	use tonic formulas to build up
STRESS	Adrenal/Fatigue Formula	meditation, walking and deep breathing are important
LOW IMMUNE FUNCTION	Immune Deficiency Formula	eliminate immune-suppressive habits (negative emotions) and drugs

SUPPORTING THERAPY:

Conservation of energy is the heart of the issue. If you are experiencing a chronic state of low energy, it is vital to walk every day—as much as can be tolerated (up to 1-2 miles), depending on the condition of one's general health. Start with 5-15 minutes of deep breathing. Work up to an hour a day if feasible. Proper elimination is important. Do not overeat, but get a sufficient quantity of the highest quality foods—choose as few processed foods as possible. Eat greens and lightly-steamed vegetables and complex starches, such as grains and legumes. For candida or chronic fatigue syndrome, add Anti-Viral and Immune Deficiency Formulas, long-term (up to 9 months). Taking relaxing herbs can help release energy. Read positive and spiritual books; a positive and hopeful attitude is absolutely necessary for restoration of health. Participating in support groups and sharing with friends are good outlets. Practice meditation; stilling the mind for even short periods saves valuable energy, which we tend to constantly expend by worrying and thinking too much.

EYEBRIGHT
NETTLES
DONG QUAI

HAY FEVER/ALLERGIES FORMULA

A formula for reducing the symptoms of allergies to airborne irritants such as pollen.

INGREDIENTS: Nettles tops, Eyebright herb, Dong Quai root, Cleavers herb, Golden seal rhizome and root, Licorice root, Mugwort herb
Liquid form

Nettles herb, Licorice root, Dong quai root, Lemon thyme herb, Eyebright herb, Golden seal rhizome and root
Caplet form

USES: For balancing the body's response to airborne irritants such as pollen, itchy eyes, runny nose, sneezing, etc.

This formula has consistently shown excellent results for helping to reduce the unpleasant symptoms of hay fever. Hay Fever Formula works in several ways to lower allergic substances in the body (dong quai, nettles),[40],[41] soothe irritation (licorice, golden seal),[42],[43] remove congestion (eyebright) and excess water (cleavers), helping to balance body systems that are affected by airborne irritants.

Urtica dioica

ENERGY: Cooling, slightly drying.

ACTIONS: Specific with slight tonic properties—calms immune overreactivity to allergens; anti-inflammatory; removes excess water. Symptomatic relief from hay fever, runny nose, itchy eyes, etc.

DOSE: One dropperful in warm water as needed up to 5x/day; or one caplet 3x/day.

CAUTIONS: Not for use for over 10 days with pre-existing deficiency or immune suppression, unless immune tonic formulas are added.

PROGRAMS: Try using it in combination with Respiratory Formula for prevention and shortening of symptoms of hay fever. For chronic deficiency, add Adrenal/Fatigue Formula (recommended) or Immune Deficiency Formula. With poor digestion or suspected food allergies, add Bitters Formula or Liver/Digestive Formula.

SUPPORTING THERAPY:

Hay fever can be a difficult problem. Keep processed fats and other refined foods to a minimum (especially any refined oils, such as margarine), choosing only high-quality whole foods such as grains, legumes, vegetables, at least one serving of steamed green vegetables a day. Extra seaweed in the diet is sometimes helpful. Determine if food allergens are adding a burden to the immune system or helping to over-sensitize it. Eliminate one of the main allergens from the diet on a trial basis for two weeks to determine if this may be a factor. The most common allergens are meat, pasteurized dairy products, wheat, and eggs. Try making a light salt solution (1/2 tsp salt to 1/2 cup water) added to golden seal tea to spray the nasal passages using an old nasal spray bottle. This may help to "wash" away pollens and other irritants before they can become allergenic.

HEADACHE FORMULA

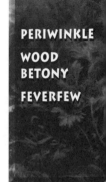

PERIWINKLE
WOOD
BETONY
FEVERFEW

INGREDIENTS: Wood Betony herb, Feverfew herb, Passion Flower herb, Periwinkle herb, Lavender oil
Liquid form

USES: For the symptomatic relief of tension headaches. Can be taken preventatively when tension headaches are a problem or are anticipated.

An herbal formula to help ease the discomfort of tension headaches. In general, the liquid form is the most rapidly absorbed and acting of any herbal preparation, and consequently is an excellent way to achieve fast headache relief. Periwinkle herb causes an increase in the blood supply to the brain in laboratory tests and was recommended by the Renaissance herbalists to cure headache.[38] This herb has proven to be a very effective one in practice to help reduce symptoms of mild tension headaches. Wood betony has a long history as a tonic herb for headaches. Passion flower and other nervous system herbs are chosen to help bring a state of relaxation, lessening the tension that can create or worsen a headache.[39]

ENERGY: Cool.

ACTIONS: Specific—increases blood flow to brain, reduces allergic/inflammatory response, relaxes mind and nervous system.

DOSE: One to two dropperfuls as needed—no more than 8 dropperfuls maximum in a day.

CAUTIONS: Follow directions, and do not use more than 4 times in a day.

PROGRAMS:

CONDITION	FORMULAS TO ADD	ADDITIONAL COMMENTS
POOR SLEEP	Sleep Formula	deep breathing and stretching before bed are helpful
NERVOUSNESS, TENSION	Relaxing Formula	deep breathing, meditation, stress-release techniques are important for lasting success
POOR DIGESTION, EMOTIONAL STRESS, LIVER INVOLVEMENT	Liver/Digestive Formula	allow at least 2 hours after eating before retiring
WEAKNESS, FATIGUE	Adrenal/Fatigue Formula, Immune Deficiency Formula	general deficiency often accompanies sleeping difficulties —it's important to build up generally with tonic formulas
MENSTRUATION	PMS/Hormonal Formula, Women's Bloodbuilder Formula	a diet rich in lightly cooked vegetables, greens, grains and legumes (with fish and chicken where there is severe deficiency) is essential

SUPPORTING THERAPY:

Stretching and massage are two great ways to keep the blood flowing into the head. If one is experiencing eyestrain, such as with computer work, stop frequently to massage the neck using strong kneading strokes. Push the thumb under the occipital ridge (the bottom back of the skull) and work along it until a sore spot is located. Try to work it out. Tension in the shoulders can also cause a reflex blood restriction. Massage of the big toes sometimes will bring relief. Pressing on the roof of the mouth with the tongue firmly for up to a minute at a time will often be effective. Using cold and hot compresses alternating on the back of the neck and skull is another good technique. If the headache is brought on by eyestrain, palm the eyes, pressing lightly for 30 seconds, then releasing. Try squeezing the eyes shut in an exaggerated way and then open them as wide as possible and hold for 10 seconds. Alternate this exercise for a few rounds. Simply shut the eyes and rest them every so often. If the mind is over-active, try meditating for 5 minutes to start. Be consistent.

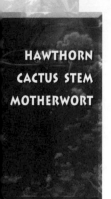

HEART AND VASCULAR TONIC FORMULA

INGREDIENTS: Hawthorn flower, Cactus stem, Motherwort herb, Chinese Sage root, Hawthorn fruit, Polygala root, Ginger oil *Liquid form*

USES: Benefits and strengthens the heart in mild to moderate heart conditions; it is safe and can be taken concurrently with many heart medications.

Hawthorn is the best-known herb for the heart and cardiovascular system throughout Europe. Modern studies and clinical reports show that it can benefit the heart by bringing more blood into the muscle itself, while steadying the heartbeat, helping to lower blood pressure, and prevent clotting. It is generally considered safe with pharmaceutical heart preparations. Cactus is an excellent cardiotonic and mild stimulant; motherwort is used in both western and Asian herbal medicine to strengthen the heart; polygala benefits the heart, according to Traditional Chinese Medicine; and Chinese sage root and ginger help to move the blood and increase oxygen and nutrient flow to the tissues.

Crataegus laevigata

ENERGY: Warm.

ACTIONS: Tonic + specific—moves the blood, increases blood flow to the heart muscle, regulates heart beat.

DOSE: 2-3 dropperfuls daily (2 in the morning, 1 in the evening), or more as needed.

CAUTIONS: It may slightly potentiate heart stimulants like digitalis (simply use a lower dose, which is preferable because of the high potential for side effects from the pharmaceutical).

PROGRAMS: For nervousness, add Relaxing Formula; for sleeplessness, add Sleep Formula; for depression, add Anti-Depression Formula; for digestive problems, such as gas, add Digestion/Bitters Formula and Liver/ Digestive Formula.

SUPPORTING THERAPY:

A low-fat, high fiber diet is a must; eliminate red meat, focus on fish and chicken; 70-80% vegetables, fruits, and grains; stress-release techniques are vital—meditation, walking, deep breathing, group counseling work, etc.

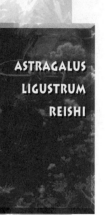

ASTRAGALUS
LIGUSTRUM
REISHI

IMMUNE DEFICIENCY (CHRONIC) FORMULA

A deeply strengthening immune support formula

INGREDIENTS: Astragalus root, Ligustrum fruit, Reishi, Shiitake, Echinacea root, North American Reishi mushroom   *Liquid form*

Astragalus root, Ligustrum fruit, Codonopsis root, Atractylodes rhizome, Reishi mushroom, Shiitake mushroom, Echinacea root and tops *Caplet form*

USES: Long-term, for strengthening the body's powers of defense or recuperation. As part of an entire program for immune imbalances such as candida infections, chronic fatigue syndrome, HIV, cancers, or other chronic viral infections and auto-immune imbalances, such as environmental allergies. For frequent colds or chronic respiratory problems.

This combination is designed to strengthen the "deep" immune system—what the Chinese call a "Chi Tonic" and western medicine a "bone marrrow reserve builder". It contains many herbs, such as astragalus,[44] reishi, and shiitake, that science has shown to have amazing immune-strengthening properties. The "power mushrooms" (reishi and shiitake)[45],[46],[47] are traditional remedies revered for their ability to enhance our natural powers of defense.

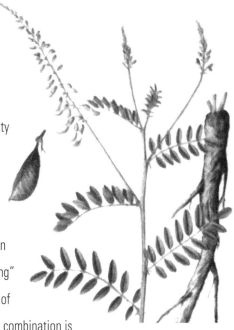

Astragalus membranaceous

Similar strengthening combinations have been used in China under the name "Fu-Zheng" therapy for perhaps thousands of years.[48] Astragalus/ligustrum combination is for long-term weakness, chronic illness, or deficiency. Many degenerative ailments, such as cancer, fall into this category. Also to be used for general immune weakness for a long period of time (3-6 months).

ENERGY: Sweet, warm, tonifying.

ACTIONS: Tonic—supports and strengthens bone-marrow reserve and immune potential. In TCM, strengthens the spleen, lung, and kidney systems.

DOSE: 25-40 drops in warm water 2-3X/day; 1X/day for maintenance; or one caplet 2x/day.

CAUTIONS: Use with Anti-Inflammatory Formula or Colds/Infections Formula in the acute phase for infections, colds, and flu. Warming immune formulas might support the pathogenic energy (bacteria, etc.) during the acute phase if used by itself in some individuals.

PROGRAMS: During the acute phase of infections, use with Colds/Infections Formula. In severe immune deficient conditions, especially when stress is a factor, add Adrenal/Fatigue Formula. For cancers, add Blood Purifier Formula. For digestive weakness, add Digestion/Bitters Formula; for coldness, add a ginseng or astragalus single-herb extract. For depression, add Anti-Depression Formula; for poor sleep, add Sleep Formula; for anxiety and nervousness, add Relaxing Formula. Take with an Adrenal/Stress Formula during times of stress. Add an Echinacea Formula and garlic when there is an acute infection. Effective when used in a program with Colds/Infections Formula and Adrenal/ Stress Formula for extra activity, though Immune Deficiency Formula contains just the right amount of echinacea for long-term use and is complete in itself.

SUPPORTING THERAPY:

Choose only the highest quality whole foods. Superfoods such as spirulina, chlorella, and barley grass offer good support. Our immune system is a direct reflection of our total health, encompassing spirit, mind, and body. Creating true health is a journey that is at times best taken with help. Realizing that we need help and asking for it are the first steps in this process. Read books on the subject, attend classes— reach out to people. Many positive new books are available now, especially on how our mind and attitude and self-acceptance can affect our health,[49,50] as well as many natural ways to build a strong body.[51]

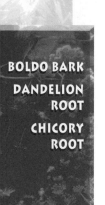

BOLDO BARK
DANDELION ROOT
CHICORY ROOT

LIVER CLEANSING FORMULA

INGREDIENTS: Boldo bark, Dandelion root & leaf, Chicory root, Lemon juice powder, Fennel seed, Oregon grape root, Cyperus, Fringe-tree (*Chionanthus*), Yellow dock, Zedoary

USES: Cleansing programs, exposure to liver toxins, acne, headaches due to "liver fire rising," emotional swings due to stagnant liver energy, symptoms associated with Pre-Menstrual Syndrome (PMS).

The liver is the most important cleansing organ in the body. It also produces bile, which emulsifies fats and aids in their absorption and assimilation. When the liver energy or "Qi" is stagnant (not moving properly), such symptoms as headache, blood-shot eyes, emotional swings (such as anger rising up or sadness that we hold onto) can ensue. The liver also breaks down hormones, such as testosterone and estrogen, causing them to build up and increase the levels beyond what is optimum, leading to symptoms of PMS and emotional swings, among others.

Cichorium intybus

ENERGY:	Cool; enters the liver channel.
ACTIONS:	Cleansing, bile-stimulating, improves fat digestion.
DOSE:	1-2 dropperfuls in a little water, ginger tea, or fennel tea 2-3 times daily before meals.
CAUTIONS:	Do not use during pregnancy, or with internal coldness and deficiency.
PROGRAMS:	For extra strength, add Digestion/Bitters Formula.

LIVER/DIGESTIVE FORMULA

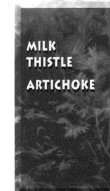

**MILK
THISTLE
ARTICHOKE**

| INGREDIENTS: | Milk Thistle seed, Artichoke leaf, Dandelion root, Turmeric rhizome, Skullcap herb, California Coast Sage herb   *Liquid form* |
| USES: | First and foremost, a digestive aid. Indicated for poor or painful digestion, gas and bloating, poor assimilation of nutrients, hepatitis, cirrhosis, general toxicity of the body; weak, sore, or congested liver, high-fat diet with poor assimilation of fats, previous bouts of hepatitis, as well as for constipation. |

It is used as a general tonic to increase the smooth functioning of the liver. Of course, with liver disease it is best to work with a competent health professional. PMS and low energy are also indications.

The ancients didn't call it the "live-r" for nothing. Some of its important functions include storing and making glucose available for energy, detoxification (including environmental poisons), storing vitamins, manufacturing immune substances, and breaking down excess hormones. It was considered by the ancients to be the seat of emotions. For more details, see my *Natural Liver Therapy*.[13]

The combination of milk thistle,[14,15,16] artichoke leaves[17,18] dandelion root,[19,20] artemisia leaf,[21] turmeric,[22] and skullcap[23] herb constitutes a powerful formula that is "energy balanced"; that is, it is neither too hot nor too cold, energetically speaking. These herbs have been shown in clinical trials and laboratory tests to help speed liver regeneration,[24] as well as enhance the secretion of bile and other digestive enzymes. These extra enzymes can help with fat, protein, and starch digestion.[25]

ENERGY: Cool, cleansing.

ACTIONS: Stimulates bile production, invigorates digestive system energy, supports liver function, protectant, regenerative.

DOSE: One dropperful in warm water or tea before meals, morning and evening, or as needed, during times of uncomfortable or weak digestion or gas. Take for up to 10 days, then take a 3 day break, then take another course of 10 days. This can be repeated, as needed. If the digestive disturbance continues for more than 30-45 days, it is best to seek a total program from a qualified health practitioner.

CAUTIONS: For deficient, cold constitutions add drops to ginger tea.

PROGRAMS: For additional digestive activation, use with Digestion/Bitters Formula; for deficiency, use with Immune Deficiency Formula and Adrenal/Fatigue Formula; with constipation, add Laxative/Bowel Tonic Formula.

SUPPORTING THERAPY:

Watch food combinations; especially inadvisable are proteins and sweet foods at the same meal, such as meat and fruit. This enhances fermentation in the colon. Acidophilus supplementation, ginger caplets, ginger tea, or liquid extract of ginger can be helpful in this case. Light exercise, such as a walk in the fresh air after meals, is advisable. Try eating a grain/fruit meal in the morning (muesli soaked in apple juice, or with yogurt), several light snacks during the day (vegetables, fruit, crackers, nut butters, etc.), and the large protein meal in the evening after working. At day's end, the mind and body should be at rest, allowing the digestion to receive more energy. A good bitter tonic formula in liquid form before big meals each day, preferably containing gentian, artichoke, and ginger is also recommended. Try adding 20 drops of Liver/ Digestive Formula to Digestion/Bitters Formula.

For liver imbalances (symptoms of headaches, depression and anger, menstrual irregularities), eliminate processed fats from the diet (extra virgin olive oil is the best), eat lots of steamed green vegetables, if tolerated, and super foods such as spirulina, a high source of easily-assimilated protein that causes little putrefaction.

MULLEIN
LEAF
RED ROOT
RED CLOVER

LYMPHATIC CLEANSER/ACTIVATOR

INGREDIENTS: Mullein leaf, Red Root, Red Clover flower, Scrophularia root, Burdock root, Ocotillo bark, Echinacea root, Myrrh oil, Ginger oil
Liquid form

USES:	Acne, dermatitis, psoriasis, cleansing programs to improve overall health during or after infections to clear the lymph of dead pathogens, immune cells, and their by-products.

Lymphatic cleansers are often added to cleansing programs for skin problems such as acne. Mullein leaf and scrophularia work on the lymph nodes and lymphatic system in the upper part of the body, ocotillo bark and red root in the lower part. Burdock is a bile stimulant and liver cleanser, echinacea is an immune stimulant, a lymphatic cleanser, and blood purifier. Myrrh oil and ginger oil help move and disperse stagnant conditions in the lymph and blood systems.

ENERGY:	Neutral, dispersing.
ACTIONS:	Specific—activates immune function, remove congestion from lymph.
DOSE:	2-3 dropperfuls 2-3 x daily as needed.
CAUTIONS:	None noted.
PROGRAMS:	For extra liver elimination, add Liver/ Digestive Formula; for extra immune stimulation, add Colds/Infections Formula; for immune support, add Immune Deficiency Formula; for adrenal support, add Adrenal/Stress Formula.

SUPPORTING THERAPY:

This formula works best with a full lymphatic massage and the liver flush for up to 7-10 days; eat a light diet consisting of mostly fresh fruits and vegetables, or combine with a 3 or 7-day fast, depending on experience and need.

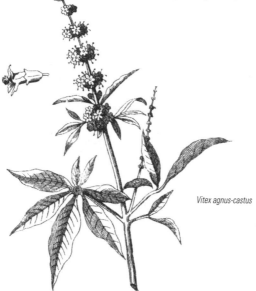

Vitex agnus-castus

MENOPAUSE FORMULA

VITEX
BLACK COHOSH
RHIZOME

INGREDIENTS: Vitex fruit, Black Cohosh rhizome and root, Date seed, Zizyphus seed, Valerian rhizome and root, Fu Ling sclerotium, Dong Quai root, Peony root, Aletris root, Tangerine oil, Lavender oil, Valerian oil
Liquid form

Vitex fruit, Black cohosh rhizome and root,
Date seed, Valerian rhizome and root, Fu Ling
sclerotium, Peony root, Tangerine oil,
Lavender oil, Valerian oil
Caplet form

USES: Helps relieve the symptoms of menopause—
vaginal dryness, hot flashes, sugar cravings,
lowered sexual drive, emotional swings
such as depression.

Peony is one of the most famous strengthening herbal tonics in Chinese
Medicine, taken by men and women. It is especially famous for women
who are weak or blood deficient, or who are having menstrual problems.
During menopause, the blood often becomes deficient, and peony (and the
herb rehmannia) works to build up strong blood and moisten organs and
tissues that might become too dry. Vitex is recommended for the same
uses by Hippocrates (455 B.C.), the famous Greek physician. It is the best
hormonal balancer, especially for promoting progesterone and restoring
healthy estrogen levels. It helps with emotional swings, food cravings,
headaches, constipation, cramps, excessive/deficient flow of menstruation.
Helps relieve undesirable feelings and symptoms during menopause.

Black cohosh is a favorite women's herb in Native American herbalism,
as well as in Eclectic medicine. The herb is traditionally used for
increasing tone to all the female organs, bringing on the menstrual
flow if it is late (emmenagogue), and relieving pain during menstruation.
Black cohosh is generally relaxing and is traditionally used to reduce pain

and inflammation of arthritis. Modern studies show that several active fractions block estrogen stimulation of the uterus and lower luteinizing hormone levels, benefiting PMS-like syndromes and symptoms of menopause. Date seed is reported to have small amounts of natural estrogen, zizyphus supports the nerves, valerian calms and relaxes, fu ling strengthens the digestion, aletris is a Native American tonic for women, and the 3 essential oils are relaxing and lift the spirits.

ENERGY: Warm.

ACTIONS: Tonic with slight specific properties— moves the blood, removes congestion, activates hormones (especially progesterone), regulates the emotions, removes stagnation from the liver.

DOSE: 1-3 dropperfuls or one caplet 2 x daily, morning and evening.

CAUTIONS: Do not take during pregnancy or when taking birth-control pills.

PROGRAMS: For depression, add Anti-Depression Formula; for sleeplessness, add Sleep Formula; for anxiety, add Relaxing Formula.

SUPPORTING THERAPY:

A diet high in soy products (tofu, tempeh) and rice, with lightly sauteed or steamed vegetables is recommended.

MOUTH CARE / GINGIVITIS / MOUTH FRESHENER FORMULA

PROPOLIS
PEPPERMINT
ECHINACEA
ROOT

A Mouth-Care Formula and Refreshing Mouth Rinse

INGREDIENTS: Echinacea root, Golden seal rhizome and root, Usnea herb, Ginger rhizome, Licorice root, Bloodroot, Propolis, Peppermint oil
Liquid Form

USES: Gingivitis, plaque preventative, receding gums, cold sores, breath freshener.

Bloodroot extract has been shown in scientific studies to protect the teeth and gums against disease-promoting bacteria. It is an ingredient in commercial mouthwash preparations.[52] Other herbs such as propolis and golden seal are astringent and anti-bacterial and help to strengthen and protect gums.[53] Echinacea and usnea help the body resist bacterial infection.[54] Ginger is warming, bringing extra blood to the gums[55] (lack of circulation is a major cause of gum disease), and the essential oils are warming and anti-bacterial. Mouth-Care Formula is a pleasant-tasting daily oral-hygiene preparation that is made entirely from herbs, distilled water, and grain alcohol—no synthetic chemicals are added.

ENERGY: Spicy warm.

ACTIONS: Specific + tonic—inhibits bacterial growth and plaque formation, stimulates blood flow to the gums, refreshes and deodorizes the breath. Excellent for gingivitis, cold sores, and as a plaque fighter.

DOSE: 10-15 drops in water as a rinse. Squirt a half-dropperful into the mouth and swish with a little water after meals. Dentists recommend brushing after every meal to prevent plaque build-up. If you can't brush, try Mouth-Care Formula. In the evening, apply a few drops to a soft-bristle brush and massage into the gums right at the gum-line. You may be surprised and pleased at the lack of plaque at your next check-up!

CAUTIONS: Large amounts undiluted may cause irritation in sensitive individuals.

PROGRAMS: As a daily rinse and application to the gums for increased oral health. Apply full-strength during times of extra irritation or infection. Mouth-Care Formula is an effective plaque fighter! Simply place a few drops on a soft-bristle brush and massage into the gum line before going to bed. After using Mouth-Care Formula for several months as a plaque preventative, it will be found that there is much less plaque build-up, as can be proven

during the next dental checkup or cleaning—
or by using plaque disclosure tablets.
For cold sores, apply directly. With mouth
infections, use echinacea or propolis
topically and echinacea internally to boost
immune response.

SUPPORTING THERAPY:

The two major factors in maintaining health
of the gums and teeth are ample blood
supply and proper hygiene. Proper blood
supply can be maintained by regularly
massaging the jaw—especially the lower
jaw. We often carry considerable tension
in the jaw area, which can lead to restricted
blood flow. Carefully (but thoroughly)
massage around any sore teeth at least
morning and evening. Rinsing with very cold
water for 30 seconds will bring a good blood
supply into the gums. Good hygiene means
brushing immediately after each meal with
a soft-bristle brush (or at least swishing
vigorously with an herbal rinse) and flossing
thoroughly at the end of the day.

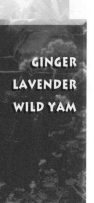

GINGER
LAVENDER
WILD YAM

NAUSEA / MORNING SICKNESS / MOTION SICKNESS FORMULA

INGREDIENTS: Ginger rhizome, Lavender blossoms, Wild yam, Tangerine peel, Magnolia bark, Fermented leaven, Ginger oil, Peppermint oil   *Caplet form*

USES: Nausea due to car, airplane, or boat travel, and all other types of motion sickness. Beneficial during pregnancy for morning sickness. May be of benefit for gas in the intestine, especially due to fermentation of vegetable foods.

Ginger has been shown to allay nausea in cases of motion sickness, reducing the tendency of vomiting and dizziness.[58] Ginger has undergone clinical trials and was shown to be more effective than dramamine in preventing and shortening nausea due to motion sickness.[59] This combination also warms the digestive tract and promotes good digestion. Lavender has been traditionally used to prevent nausea,[60] and wild yam is antispasmodic, reducing the tendency of the muscles of the digestive tract to cramp, recommended by herbalists to help alleviate nausea.[61]

ENERGY: Spicy warm, aromatic.

ACTIONS: Specific + stimulating tonic—anti-nauseant, warming, stimulating to the digestion, uplifting to the spirits.

DOSE: 1-2 caplets as needed. Ginger/lavender combination normally begins to be effective about 10-20 minutes after it is taken. As a preventive for motion sickness, take 1/2 hour before journey.

CAUTIONS: For excess heat conditions/constitutions use sparingly (no more than 1-2 caplets for up to 1 or 2 days).

PROGRAMS: When excited or apprehensive about traveling or other emotional issues, try taking this formula with a relaxing one, such as Relaxing Formula. For extra digestive stimulation and to cool down the formula, add Liver/Digestive Formula; for a warm blood purification formula, add Blood Purifier Formula to warm it up.

SUPPORTING TREATMENT:

Slow, regular breathing, focusing on the breath is also helpful. When overheated, try applying cool compresses to the forehead. Apply pressure to the back of the hand between the base of the thumb and 1st finger, "working out" any sore spots.

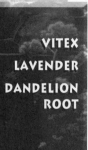

PMS / HORMONAL FORMULA

INGREDIENTS: Vitex fruit, Dandelion root, Black Cohosh rhizome and root, Blue Cohosh rhizome and root, Cramp bark, Prickly Ash bark, Lavender oil *Liquid form*

Vitex fruit, Cramp bark, Dandelion root, Prickly Ash bark, Blue cohosh root, Valerian rhizome and root, Lavender oil *Caplet form*

USES: For PMS-like symptoms, cramps, depression, excessive flow, irregular cycles, fibroid cysts, increases milk flow after birth, adolescent acne.

German scientists have shown that the star herb, Vitex, works through the pituitary gland to regulate proper female hormonal function. This results in a smoother and more symptom-free menstrual period.[56] Other herbs are known by herbalists to nourish and tonify the uterus. Black cohosh is a stimulating tonic, blue cohosh a nutritive tonic, and cramp bark is used traditionally by herbalists to help relieve uterine cramps.[57] Lavender essential oil is added for its aromatherapy benefits and has long been thought to lift the spirits.

Cimicifuga racemosa

Because excess estrogen can enhance symptoms associated with PMS, proper liver health is vital during the cycle, as it is the liver's job to remove excess estrogen from the body. For this reason, dandelion is added to the formula. In recent German studies, black cohosh has been shown to block the overstimulation of estrogen on estrogen-sensitive tissues, as well as slowing its overproduction by reducing luteinizing hormone (LH) production. Women's Hormone Balancing Formula is used where PMS is a problem, or to regulate and tone the female generative function, generally.

ENERGY: Warm.

ACTIONS: Stimulating tonic + specific—warms, moves blood, regulates hormones; relaxes, tones uterus; lifts spirits.

DOSE: 1 dropperful in warm water 3X/day starting 4 days before the onset of the menstrual flow. Take 1 dropper morning and evening during the flow and for 3 days following. For maintenance, long-term, use 1 dropperful before breakfast. (2 dropperfuls = 1 caplet)

CAUTIONS: Vitex products are reported (in Germany) to possibly alter the way birth-control pills (containing progesterone) affect the body. In my opinion, this may not be significant in terms of the efficacy of birth-control pills to prevent pregnancy, but the possibility of some effect should be watched for.

PROGRAMS: Take 1 dropperful 3X/day for up to 8 months and add castor oil packs daily for 45 minutes in the evening for as long as needed. For adolescent acne in males, take 1 dropper 2X/day along with Acne Formula.

CONDITION	FORMULAS TO ADD	ADDITIONAL COMMENTS
DEPRESSION	Anti-Depression Formula, Brain Formula	with coldness, take in ginger tea
SUGAR CRAVINGS	Bitters/Digestion Formula	be strict about avoiding any simple sugars (honey, maple syrup, fruit juices, etc.); substitute whole grains, stevia, licorice tea
EMOTIONAL SWINGS	Liver/Digestive Formula	take drops in rosemary or lavender tea
POOR SLEEP	Sleep Formula	stretching and deep breathing help
ANXIETY	Relaxing Formula	meditation and deep breathing are helpful
FATIGUE	Women's Bloodbuilder Formula, Energy/Fatigue Formula, Ten Ginsengs Formula, and Adrenal/Fatigue Formula	eat mostly cooked foods; some fish or chicken may be desirable

SUPPORTING THERAPY:

Mild exercise is of great help to increase elimination, but proper rest is also important. A short period of deep breathing can be of value. Massage the pelvic area to help relieve congestion. Light nourishing meals can assist the body in one of its main functions during the menstrual flow—elimination.

RELAXING FORMULA

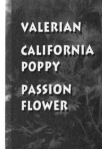

VALERIAN
CALIFORNIA
POPPY
PASSION
FLOWER

INGREDIENTS: Valerian rhizome and root, California poppy plant, Passion flower herb, Hops strobiles, Hawthorn flower   *Liquid form*

Valerian rhizome and root, California poppy plant, Passion flower herb, Catnip herb, Valerian oil   *Caplet form*

USES: Nervousness, sleeplessness, restlessness, anxiety, tight muscles (or anytime a natural herbal relaxing preparation is needed).

Herbal sedative and relaxing formulas on the market commonly use dried herbs, but many herbalists feel that passion flower, valerian, and hops, three of the most popular relaxing herbs, lose potency when dried. This combination is formulated from fresh or fresh-dried herbs. Valerian helps relieve emotional stress and nervousness and

causes a more relaxed night's sleep.[62]
Passion flower is used for mental tranquility,[63]
and California poppy[64] is commonly used in
Europe as an excellent relaxing herb and
antispasmodic, yet safe enough for children.
Hawthorn has been shown in European
clinical trials to possess
calming activity.[65]

Valeriana officinalis

ENERGY:	Warm, bitter.
ACTIONS:	Specific + stimulating tonic—calms nervous system, relaxes, helps allay anxiety, promotes sound sleep.
DOSE:	One to two dropperfuls or caplets as needed. For stress and anxiety take through out the day. For sleep problems take at bedtime.
CAUTIONS:	May cause slight headache if used in high doses (over 2-3 dropperfuls in sensitive individuals).
PROGRAMS:	For internal coldness, add Digestion/Bitters Formula; for deficient states, add Adrenal/ Fatigue Formula and Immune Deficiency Formula; for depression, add Anti-Depression

Formula; for mild cardiovascular problems, add Heart Formula; for menstrual difficulties, add PMS/Hormonal Formula or Women's Bloodbuilder Formula; for difficult sleep problems, add Sleep Formula; for menopause, add Menopause Formula. If taken during the day, the preparation does not normally induce drowsiness.

SUPPORTING TREATMENT:

Try a short, relaxing walk before bedtime. Five or ten minutes of stretching can be amazingly effective for bringing on the sleep response. Meditate by concentrating on the breath. Begin with 5 minutes a day before bed or during times of stress. Make sure to take a cool shower or bath after every hot or warm one. This has a very strengthening offect on the nerves; excessive hot water can weaken the nerves.

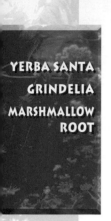

RESPIRATORY / ASTHMA / CONGESTION FORMULA

A warming respiratory tract stimulant formula

INGREDIENTS: Yerba santa herb, Grindelia flower buds, Marshmallow root, Tangerine peel, Golden seal rhizome and root, Poplar leaf buds, Licorice root, Usnea herb, Cayenne fruit
Liquid form

USES: Congestion due to colds, flu, bronchitis, asthma and other respiratory infections, and hay fever allergies.

The two star herbs in this traditional combination are western herbs that were formerly "official" in the U.S. Pharmacopoeia (grindelia and yerba santa).[66] They are known to have warming, anti-bacterial, and expectorant qualities.[67] Marshmallow root[68] and licorice[69] are soothing and anti-inflammatory herbs to help soothe irritated mucous membranes. Golden seal helps strengthen mucous membranes and is used traditionally as a cooling herb to remove heat during infection.[70] Tangerine peel is a traditional Chinese herb for strengthening lungs,[71] and it adds flavor and sweetness to the formula, as does licorice. Licorice is anti-inflammatory and is traditionally used to "harmonize" the action of herbal formulas.[72,73] Poplar (Balm of Gilead) is used by herbalists as an expectorant and anti-inflammatory herb,[74] and cayenne is a warming expectorant.[75]

This formula can be taken when there is any lung or respiratory weakness or for chronic bronchial or throat problems or asthma. It helps the body to eliminate mucus, while strengthening the respiratory tract in general.

It is also good during hay fever attacks, or other respiratory congestion, especially combined with Hay Fever/Allergies Formula.

ENERGY: Warm, spicy.

ACTIONS: Specific + slight tonic properties—warms, stimulates upper respiratory function (especially bronchial area); increases expectoration of mucus; pain-relieving, cough-relieving; anti-bacterial, anti-viral.

DOSE: 25-40 drops straight (it may be too spicy to take straight for some people), or in a little water as needed.

CAUTIONS: Use sparingly in excess heat conditions, or add golden seal.

PROGRAMS: For extra potency, add Colds/Infections Formula; for chronic conditions, with low-grade fever, add Immune Deficiency Formula. As a general strengthening aid for the upper respiratory tract, take a dropperful of Respiratory Formula in a little water and feel the warmth spread to the bronchial area.

Make a pot of garden sage and organic lemon peel tea. Add the juice of half a lemon after light simmering for 15 minutes. Add 1 dropperful of Respiratory Formula. Sip 1 cup 2-3 times a day, especially in the morning and evening. For extra soothing support, add marshmallow root and a little licorice to the tea (simmer first for 10 minutes before adding the other herbs). Try an herbal "steam" by putting eucalyptus leaves into a pot of simmering water. Turn off the heat and place a towel over the head, lean over the steaming pot and inhale repeatedly, breathing the essential oils and steam into the bronchi and lungs. This can have a very decongesting, expectorating, and clearing effect.

**VALERIAN
KAVA KAVA
LINDEN
LEAF**

SLEEP FORMULA

INGREDIENTS: Valerian rhizome, Linden leaf, Hops strobiles, Kava Kava root, Chamomile flower, Celery seed, Catnip herb, Wild Lettuce herb, Orange oil, Tangerine oil, Valerian oil   *Liquid form*

Valerian rhizome, Kava Kava root, California poppy plant, Hops strobiles, Fu ling sclerotium, Polygala root, Orange oil, Valerian oil   *Caplet form*

USES: Sleeplessness, irregular sleep patterns.

This formula includes herbs that are traditionally used to bring on a refreshing, sound sleep without creating a dull or groggy feeling the next morning. Catnip, valerian, linden, and hops are all known to be effective. Kava kava is relaxing to the body, mildly euphoric, and dream-enhancing. Chamomile is mildly relaxing to the digestive tract, celery seed is a nerve tonic, wild lettuce is known to be calming, and the three essential oils are strongly relaxing.

ENERGY: Warm.

ACTIONS: Specific + slight tonic properties—relaxes central nervous function and muscles, induces sleep.

DOSE: 2-3 dropperfuls or 1-2 caplets as needed.

CAUTIONS: Large doses (over 3-4 dropperfuls at a time) can cause headache, may lead to grogginess in the morning.

PROGRAMS: For extra relaxation potential, add Relaxing Formula; for depression, add Anti-Depression Formula; for painful or weak digestion, add Digestion/Bitters Formula and Liver/Digestive Formula.

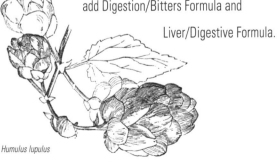

Humulus lupulus

SUPPORTING THERAPY:

Concentrate on deep breathing and relaxing. Try to eat at least 3 hours before going to bed and especially avoid any stimulating drinks.

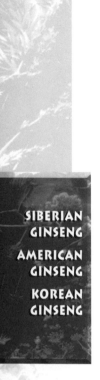

SIBERIAN GINSENG
AMERICAN GINSENG
KOREAN GINSENG

TEN GINSENGS FORMULA

INGREDIENTS: Siberian Ginseng root, American Ginseng root, Korean Ginseng root, Prince's Ginseng root, Glehnia root, Codonopsis root, Chinese Ginseng root, Ginseng leaf, White Chinese Ginseng root, Tienchi Ginseng root, Tangerine peel, Ginger rhizome
Liquid form

USES: Chronic fatigue, sexual weakness, fertility problems, coldness, poor circulation, poor digestion and assimilation.

A blend of herbs that are traditionally associated with ginseng in Traditional Chinese Medicine. Unlike a pure Panax ginseng product, this formula provides a stronger, more broad-spectrum formula that is less likely to cause over-stimulation. It can also be taken for several months as a general tonic formula to increase endurance, counteract stress, support the adrenal system, and enhance digestion.

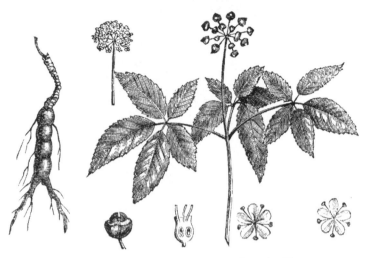

Panax quinquefolium

ENERGY: Warm.

ACTIONS: Tonic + specific—improves steroid hormone output, activates circulation, supports nerve function, relaxes nervous system, improves reproductive capabilities, nourishes vital essence.

DOSE: 1-3 dropperfuls or caplets as needed, especially in the morning.

CAUTIONS: For people who are under 40 and in good health with no fatigue, use sparingly; not recommended for people with heat conditions, such as chronic headaches.

PROGRAMS: With lowered sexual desire, use with Aphrodisiac Formula; for nervousness or sleeplessness, add Relaxing Formula; for

weak digestion, add Digestion/Bitters
Formula or Liver/Digestive Formula; for
depression, add Anti-Depression Formula.

SUPPORTING THERAPY:

A healthful diet and life-style should
be followed to constantly improve the
level of health.

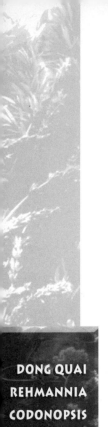

DONG QUAI
REHMANNIA
CODONOPSIS

WOMEN'S BLOODBUILDER FORMULA

INGREDIENTS: Dong quai root, Rehmannia root, Codonopsis
root, Fu ling sclerotium, Peony root,
Atractylodes rhizome, Ligusticum root,
Licorice root, Yellow dock root, Nettles herb,
Food grown iron   *Caplet form*

USES: Anemia, fatigue, depression, pallor
due to deficiency of blood.

Blood tonics have been popular In all traditional systems of healing.
In Traditional European Medicine (TEM), iron tonics, sometimes with the
addition of high-iron or other synergistic herbs such as nettles or yellow
dock, have been available for many centuries. Floradix herbal iron is a
modern example. In Traditional Chinese Medicine (TCM), blood tonics

for women and men have been an integral part of the system for several thousand years. For instance, dong quai (*Angelica sinensis*), an herb primarily recommended for its blood-tonic properties, is arguably the best-selling herb in the entire Chinese Pharmacopoeia. The famous TCM formula which contains dong quai as a lead herb, Women's Precious Pills, is one of the best-selling Chinese Patents. With this formula, I am taking the most important blood-building components from both TEM and TCM and blending them together.

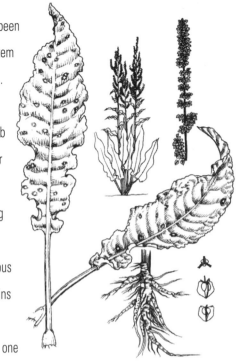

Rumex crispus

The two western herbs, nettles and yellow dock, are the most important western blood-building herbs.

ENERGY: Warm.

ACTIONS: Tonic—builds blood, strengthens spleen, improves digestion, supports adrenals, aids in assimilation of iron.

DOSE: 2 caplets 2-3 x daily.

CAUTIONS: Use sparingly during acute infections.

PROGRAMS: For immune weakness, add Immune
Deficiency Formula; for chronic fatigue,
add Adrenal/Fatigue Formula; for mild
depression, add Anti-Depression Formula;
for sleeping difficulties, add Sleep Formula;
for nervousness and mild anxiety, add
Relaxing Formula.

SUPPORTING THERAPY:
Add a variety of seaweeds and dark-green
leafy vegetables to the diet.

SINGLE HERB EXTRACTS

ASTRAGALUS

Called Huang Chi in Chinese medicine, this is one of the world's greatest immune tonics. The Chinese look at it as being a "Chi" tonic— one that increases the body's resistance and vitality of the immune system. It is a deep immune tonic that increases the "bone marrow reserve", increasing the body's ability to produce more immune effector cells (such as t-cells), protecting us from "pathogens," or what is called in Traditional

Chinese Medicine, "pernicious influences." Astragalus is a popular remedy in China used as a daily tonic when one is not feeling well or if the constitution is weak. Astragalus has a sweet nature, as do most tonic herbs.[78],[79]

In liquid form. High grade.

BLACK WALNUT

Black walnut is an astringent herb that is used for diarrhea. Because of its high tannin content, it has also been used internally as an anthelmintic and externally for ringworm. It is an excellent traveling companion in areas where water and food may contain bacteria or parasites, leading to gastrointestinal symptoms such as nausea, abdominal pains, and diarrhea. Use as a preventative (1-2 dropperfuls several times daily).

In liquid form.

DANDELION

The root of the common dandelion of lawns and gardens is a widely-used herb for cooling and cleansing the liver. Use it in tea form (add 2 dropperfuls of the liquid extract to a little ginger tea) to help with headaches, emotional swings during menstruation, acne, mood swings, and other problems related to "liver heat."

In liquid form.

DONG QUAI

Dong Quai (*Angelica sinensis*), an herb primarily recommended for its blood-tonic properties, is arguably the best-selling herb in the entire Chinese Pharmacopoeia. The famous TCM formula, Women's Precious Pills, (which contains Dong Quai as a lead herb), is one of the best-selling Chinese Patents. Dong quai vitalizes the blood and is tonic to the uterus and female generative organs.

In liquid form.

FEVERFEW

The common garden feverfew is popularly used in England and other parts of Europe for its anti-inflammatory properties. It is recommended for migraine headaches (take 2 dropperfuls of the liquid extract every day for up to 5 months as a fair trial to see if it can help). It is also recommended for inflammatory types of arthritis. There are at least two double-blind studies to support its effectiveness.

In liquid form.

GINGER, HAWAIIAN

An excellent herb for supporting digestion, relieving nausea (from any cause, including motion sickness and morning sickness), and generally stimulating circulation. Extensively used in Chinese and western herbal formulas. Ginger has been used in Europe throughout the ages to alleviate painful digestion, flatulence, colic, and diarrhea and as an ingredient in bitters formulas. Often added to laxative herbs to prevent "griping" or intestinal spasms. In liquid form.

GINKGO

One of the most interesting herbs of the last few years. Improves brain function, including memory and alertness. Protects blood vessels, improves circulation, and is a powerful antioxidant. Best herb for ringing in the ears (tinnitis).
In liquid and caplet form.

GINSENG

Woods-grown American ginseng is planted in its natural habitat and monitored but has no fertilizers or fungicides applied to it. The panacea herb of ancient China. Excellent for people over 50 to improve vital energy, sexual energy, and enhance digestive powers. Often blended with other herbs in formulas. American ginseng is more supportive to the adrenals and not as stimulating as Chinese ginseng. Its use is more appropriate for young people and can be taken for longer periods of time (up to several months).

In liquid and caplet form.

GOLDEN SEAL

This North American native herb is widely known and used for colds, flu, and sinus infections. Lowers inflammation, helps cool infections of the mucous membranes. Useful when blended with echinacea (1 part golden seal to 3 parts echinacea).

In liquid form.

GOTU KOLA

This ancient Ayurvedic herb is thought to improve memory and mental vigor and act as an adaptogen. Externally, it is effective for burns, wounds, and ulcerated skin conditions. Gotu kola has been used as a sedative for insomnia and as an antispasmodic.

In liquid form.

HAWTHORN

The extract is well-researched and has a long history of use as the herb of choice for strengthening and protecting the cardiovascular system, especially the heart. To be used in extract form long-term, even over a number of years.

In liquid form.

KAVA KAVA

Kava is the traditional herbal beverage of the South Seas. In parts of Polynesia, it is consumed every day as a recreational drink that relaxes the body and is slightly euphoric. It is used in different cultures to relieve fatigue, possibly by relaxing and helping to provide a deep sleep. Kava has been touted for its energy-promoting and communication-enhancing effects.

In liquid form.

MILK THISTLE SEED

The seed-shell of this wonderful herb yields a group of flavonoid-like compounds, collectively called silymarin, which show remarkable virtues in restoring and maintaining liver health. In Europe, it has a centuries-old reputation and many years of scientific study. Milk Thistle is used for hepatitis, cirrhosis, any toxic condition of the liver, and by alcoholics, to protect and rebuild the liver.[80] The flavonoids bind to the cell membrane of the liver cell hepatocyte, protecting it from damage by toxic chemicals such as pesticides. It also enters the hepatocyte and speeds the production of new enzymes and proteins, so the liver actually is regenerated and restored at an increased rate.[81] It is useful also for psoriasis, according to clinical results. Wildcrafted. In liquid form.

PAU D'ARCO

Since information on its anti-fungal and anti-candida properties were made known, this South American herb, derived from a common forest tree, has been tremendously popular. It is the herb of choice for Candidiasis, an increasingly widespread disease of the last several years, due to the overuse of antibiotics and other stressors on our immune function. Scientific studies also show that the active ingredient of Pau d'arco, lapachol, can inhibit tumor growth.[82]

Pau d'arco, also called "ipe roxo," is actually the inner bark from a tree of the Bignoniaceae family, though there is some confusion about the tree's botanical identity—probably several species from the genus Tecoma or Tabebuia are used. Pau d'arco should have a rich red color and an aroma resembling vanilla. It contains quinones that are strongly antibacterial and anti-fungal.

Plantation-Grown Argentinian. In liquid form.

PROPOLIS

A natural bee product, propolis is used by the colony to seal the hives against invaders or bacteria or fungal infection. It has shown strong anti-bacterial, anti-viral, and anti-fungal properties. It is especially useful in the mouth, to prevent gum disease. Externally it can be used for any kind of infection. Internally, it counteracts urinary tract infections, respiratory infections, and it is warming and expectorant (helps remove excess mucus). There are international conferences every year where many scientific papers are delivered on the benefits of propolis. It contains flavonoids and resins as the main active compounds. [83]

Bee resin. In liquid form

REISHI

Reishi is a mushroom renowned for its powerful immune-strengthening, antiviral, and antitumor properties. This rejuvenative tonic has shown the ability to regulate blood sugar and may help lower cholesterol. It is known to protect the body against free radicals and the effects of radiation.

In liquid form.

SIBERIAN GINSENG

This herb is a member of the Ginseng family, Araliaceae, like Panax ginseng, but has a different action than Panax. Panax is considered a digestive and "chi" tonic, and Siberian Ginseng is considered the "best of the adaptogens". Panax is also warmer and more stimulating than Eleuthero. Panax is not traditionally recommended to be taken by young people (under 40) for long periods (more than a week or two), because it may be too stimulating, but it is a wonderful warming tonic for older people and can be taken on a regular basis. Eleuthero, on the other hand, can be taken regularly by both men and women of all ages. It is by far the best studied in this class of herbs, with the Russians leading the way in research. Twenty million Russian workers take "Eleuthero" (as it is also called) every day—the treatments are sponsored by the government. In studies with thousands of people, eleuthero preparations, when taken consistently, decrease sick days, increase productivity and learning, and combat fatigue. It modulates stress hormones through the 'pituitary-adrenal' axis, helping the body to adapt to non-specific stress and support-ing adrenal function.[84] It is good for blood-sugar regulation, jet-lag, chron-ic tiredness, increased endurance, and whenever a person is under stress. In liquid form.

ST. JOHN'S WORT

This common European and American weedy plant shows great promise as an antiviral and anti-inflammatory agent. It has long been used as a remedy for mild depression. St. John's wort is excellent for repairing nerve damage and reducing pain and inflammation. In liquid form.

USNEA

Usnea is known as the herbal antibiotic. In the laboratory, this common lichen has shown powerful inhibitory activity against strep, staph, and pneumonia infections. It is also good for urinary tract infections, respiratory ailments, and colds. In liquid form.

VALERIAN

Valerian is used primarily for sleeplessness, restlessness, anxiety, or tension—especially in the body (as opposed to passion flower, which relaxes the mental and emotional processes).

There are scientific studies which show it helps one fall asleep faster, by lessening the time spent trying to get comfortable and tossing and turning. It was long used for hysteria and any emotional upsets. Valerian is best when fresh or freshly-dried—look for a preparation that uses this kind of plant material, which has a finer relaxing property and not as many side effects as the long-stored dry root.[85]

Fresh root. In liquid and caplet form.

VITEX

One of the best-known women's herbs, it was recommended by Hippocrates (450 B.C.) for the same purposes as today: menstrual imbalances, hormonal difficulties (PMS, menopause), and to bring on mother's milk. Also used in larger amounts (2 dropperfuls twice daily or more) to remove uterine fibroids.

In liquid form.

WILD OATS

Wild oats is a tonifying nervine and sedative herb that is well-known for its anti-addictive effects. It strengthens the nerves and is good for insomnia due to mental exhaustion.

In liquid form.

The following recommendations are for educational and health-increasing use only and not meant to be a prescription for any disease. If you are experiencing symptoms, I always recommend contacting a qualified natural health practitioner or physician for a diagnosis and total health program.

APPENDIX: HERBAL ENERGETICS AND SYSTEMS OF HEALING

KEY TO TRADITIONAL MEDICINES

NAM - North American Medicine

TCM - Traditional Chinese Medicine

TEM - Traditional European Medicine

SAM - South American Medicine

PM - Polynesian Medicine

KEY TO HERBAL ENERGETICS

S - specific

ST - stimulating tonic

NT - nutritive tonic

HERBAL ENERGETICS AND ORIGINS OF KEY HERBS

HERB	ORIGIN	SPECIFIC	STIMULATING TONIC	NUTRITIVE TONIC
ASTRAGALUS:	TCM			NT
ATRACTYLODES:	TCM			NT
AURICULARIA:	TCM, TEM			NT
BLACK COHOSH:	NAM		ST	
BURDOCK ROOT:	NAM			NT
CACTUS:	TEM		ST	
CALIFORNIA POPPY:	NAM	S		
CASCARA SAGRADA:	NAM	S	ST	
CHAMOMILE:	TEM	S		
CHOCOLATE:	SAM	S		
CODONOPSIS:	TCM			NT
DAMIANA:	NAM	S		
ECHINACEA:	TEM, NAM	S	ST	
ELEUTHERO:	TEM			NT
EYEBRIGHT:	TEM	S		
FEVERFEW:	TEM	S		
FO-TI:	TCM			NT
FU LING: (hoelen)	TCM			NT
GENTIAN:	TCM		ST	
GINGER:	TEM, TCM		ST	
GINKGO:	TCM, TEM	S	ST	
GINSENG:	TEM, TCM			NT
GOLDEN SEAL:	TCM	S		
GOTU KOLA:	NAM			NT
GRINDELIA:	NAM	S		
HAWTHORN:	NAM			NT
KAVA KAVA:	TEM	S		

HERB	ORIGIN	SPECIFIC	STIMULATING TONIC	NUTRITIVE TONIC
LIGUSTRUM:	PM			NT
MELISSA: (lemon balm)	TEM	S		
NETTLES:	TEM	S		NT
OREGON GRAPE ROOT:	NAM	S		
PASSION FLOWER:	TEM	S		
PEONY:	TCM			NT
PERIWINKLE:	TEM	S		
PROPOLIS:	TEM	S		
RED CLOVER:	TEM	S		
RED KOREAN PANAX GINSENG:	TCM		ST	
RED ROOT:	NAM	S		
REHMANNIA:	TCM			NT
REISHI:	TCM			NT
SANDALWOOD:	TEM		ST	
SARSAPARILLA:	NAM		ST	
SCROPHULARIA ROOT:	TEM, NAM	S		NT
ST. JOHN'S WORT:	TEM	S		
TREMELLA:	NAM, TEM, TCM			NT
TURMERIC:	TEM		ST	
USNEA:	TEM, TCM	S		
VALERIAN:	TEM	S		
VITEX:	TEM	S		
WHITE MULBERRY:	TCM			NT
WHITE WILLOW BARK:	TEM	S		
WILD OATS:	TEM	S		NT
YERBA SANTA:	NAM	S	ST	
YUCCA:	NAM	S		

ENERGETICS OF HERBAL FORMULAS

HERB	SPECIFIC	STIMULATING TONIC	NUTRITIVE TONIC	USES
ACNE/SKIN FORMULA	S	ST		acne, skin rashes
ADRENAL/FATIGUE FORMULA			NT	adrenal weakness, low energy, excessive stress
ADRENAL/STRESS FORMULA			NT	jet lag, weakened adrenals, stress adaptation
ANTI-DEPRESSION FORMULA	S	ST		depression, tension, anxiety, restlessness
ANTI-INFLAMMATORY FORMULA	S			arthritis, bursitis, athletic injuries
ANTI-VIRAL FORMULA	S			AIDS, colds, flu, herpes
APHRODISIAC		ST		impotence, low sex drive
BITTERS/DIGESTION FORMULA		ST		poor digestion, bloating, lack of appetite, anemia, recovery from illness, immune weakness, fatigue
BLADDER/KIDNEY FORMULA (Urinary Tract Infections)	S	ST		cystitis, irritable bladder, mild urinary tract infections
BLOOD PURIFIER	S			acne, boils, carbuncles, dermatitis, cysts, tumors
BRAIN AND MEMORY FORMULA		ST	NT	poor memory, muddled thinking, mental fatigue
CHILDREN'S IMMUNE FORMULA	S			colds and flu; respiratory, urinary and other infections

HERB	SPECIFIC	STIMULATING TONIC	NUTRITIVE TONIC	USES
CHILDREN'S RELAXING FORMULA	S			insomnia, nervousness, stomach cramps
COLDS/INFECTIONS/ FLU FORMULA (Echinacea Golden seal Formula)	S			colds, flu, sore throat, chronic infections
ECHINACEA BLEND	S			colds and flu; respiratory, urinary, & other infections
ECHINACEA/ VITAMIN C	S			colds, flu, infections
ENERGY/FATIGUE FORMULA		ST		to enhance natural energy release; pre-exercise use
HAY FEVER/ ALLERGIES FORMULA	S			irritation from pollen
HEADACHE FORMULA	S			tension headaches
HEART & VASCULAR TONIC FORMULA		ST		heart strengthener
IMMUNE DEFICIENCY (CHRONIC) FORMULA			NT	candida, chronic fatigue, HIV, cancer, chronic viral infections
LAXATIVE/BOWEL TONIC	S			constipation, irregularity
LIVER CLEANSING FORMULA	S			exposure to liver toxins, acne, mood swings, PMS
LIVER/DIGESTIVE FORMULA	S	ST		liver congestion, acne, boils, hepatitis, painful digestion, poor fat digestion

HERB	SPECIFIC	STIMULATING TONIC	NUTRITIVE TONIC	USES
LYMPHATIC CLEANSER/ ACTIVATOR	S			acne. dermatitis, psoriasis
MENOPAUSE FORMULA		ST		vaginal dryness, hot flashes, emotional swings
MOUTH CARE / GINGIVITIS/ BREATH FRESHENER	S	ST		gum irritation or infection, to prevent plaque build-up
NAUSEA/MORNING SICKNESS / MOTION SICKNESS	S			motion sickness, morning sickness, digestion
PMS/HORMONAL FORMULA		ST		cramps, depression, fibroid cysts, to increase milk flow
RELAXING FORMULA (STRESS / NERVOUSNESS/ ANXIETY)	S			nervousness, tight muscles, sleeplessness
RESPIRATORY / ASTHMA / CONGESTION FORMULA	S	ST		flu, bronchitis, asthma, and other respiratory infections
SLEEP FORMULA	S			insomnia, irregular sleep patterns
TEN GINSENGS		ST	NT	chronic fatigue, sexual weakness, fertility problems, poor circulation
WOMEN'S BLOODBUILDER			NT	anemia

HERBAL PRESCRIBER

ABDOMINAL PAIN   Digestion/Bitters Formula,
Peppermint tea

ABSCESS   Colds/Infections Formula and Liver
Cleansing Formula, Acne Formula,
Anti-Inflammatory Formula, Blood Purifier
Formula, Lymphatic Formula

ACNE,   Acne Formula, Blood Purifier Formula,
COMMON OR CYSTIC   Lymphatic Formula, Echinacea Blend

ADRENALS, WEAK   Adrenal/Stress Formula, Adrenal/Fatigue
(adrenal insufficiency or exhaustion)   Formula, Siberian ginseng,
Ten Ginsengs Formula

ALCOHOLISM   Adrenal/Fatigue Formula,
Liver/Digestive Formula

ALLERGIES   Hay Fever Formula, Adrenal/Stress
Formula, Adrenal/Fatigue Formula,
Respiratory Formula, Anti-Inflammatory
Formula, Blood Purifier Formula

ALTERATIVE   Echinacea (concentrated), Colds/Infections
Formula, Blood Purifier Formula, Lymphatic
Formula

ALZHEIMER'S   Brain and Memory Formula

ANEMIA, SIMPLE   Women's Bloodbuilder Formula

ANGER   Liver Cleansing Formula, Liver/Digestive
Formula, Relaxing Formula

ANGINA, MILD   Hawthorn, Heart Formula

ANXIETY	Relaxing/Sleep Formula, Adrenal/Stress Formula, Adrenal/Fatigue Formula, Wild oats, Valerian
APPETITE	Adrenal/Stress Formula, Liver/Digestive Formula, Digestion/Bitters Formula, Gotu kola
ARRHYTHMIA, HEART	Heart and Vascular Tonic Formula, extra magnesium, avoid sugar
ARTHRITIS	Feverfew, Adrenal/Stress Formula, Adrenal/ Fatigue Formula, Liver Cleansing Formula
ASTHMA	Respiratory Formula, Relaxing Formula
BACK PAIN	Relaxing Formula, Sleep Formula
BITES	Echinacea (concentrated) topically; internally, Colds/Infections Formula
BLADDER, WEAK	Small amounts of Bladder/Kidney Formula (10 to 20 drops 2X/day), Saw palmetto, Kava kava
BLADDER INFECTION	Bladder/Kidney Formula, Echinacea Blend, Kava kava
BLOOD BUILDERS	Anemia Formula + superfoods, chlorophyl
BLOOD CLEANSERS	Echinacea Blend, Colds/Infections Formula, Liver Cleanser Formula, Acne/Skin Formula
BLOOD CHOLESTEROL	Liver/Digestive Formula
BLOOD POISONING	Blood Purifier Formula, Echinacea Blend, Colds/Infections Formula
BLOOD SUGAR, HIGH	Eleuthero, Adrenal/Stress Formula

BLOOD SUGAR, LOW	Eleuthero, Adrenal/Stress Formula, Adrenal/Fatigue Formula
BOILS	Echinacea, Blood Purifier Formula
BREASTS, SORE	Castor oil packs, PMS/Hormonal Formula in liquid or caplet, Vitex
BRONCHITIS	Respiratory Formula, Echinacea Blend Immune Deficiency Formula (chronic), Usnea
BRUISES	Arnica, St. John's wort oil externally
BURNS	Echinacea Blend, Calendula cream (externally), Gotu kola
CANCER	Immune Deficiency Formula, Blood Purifier Formula (best to work with a physician and qualified natural health practitioner)
CANDIDA	Immune Deficiency Formula, Black walnut, Pau d'arco, Echinacea Blend, Eleuthero, Liver/Digestive Formula, Digestion/Bitters Formula
CAR SICKNESS	Nausea Formula
CATARRH	Respiratory Formula, Echinacea Blend
CHILDBIRTH, STIM.	Blue cohosh, PMS/Hormonal Formula in liquid form
CHRONIC FATIGUE SYNDROME	Immune Deficiency Formula, Adrenal/Fatigue Formula, Energy Formula
CIRCULATION, POOR	Nausea Formula, Brain/Memory Formula

CIRRHOSIS	Milk Thistle, Liver/Digestive Formula (best to work with a physician and natural health practitioner)
COLDS	Echinacea/Vitamin C Formula, Colds/Infections Formula, Echinacea Blend, Immune Deficiency Formula
COLIC	Chamomile tea, Relaxing Formula, Sleep Formula in tea or juice
COLITIS	Relaxing Formula, Sleep Formula Chamomile tea ad lib.
COLON, TOXIC	Liver/Digestive Formula, cleansing program, colonic, light cleansing diet
CONJUNCTIVITIS	Colds/Infections Formula, Golden seal wash
CONSTIPATION	Liver/Digestive Formula, Laxative Formula
COUGH	Respiratory Formula, Relaxing Formula, Sleep Formula, Colds/Infections Formula (when there is an upper respiratory tract infection with cough)
CRAMPS, MENSTRUAL	PMS/Hormonal Formula in liquid or caplet, Relaxing Formula, Sleep Formula, Valerian
CYSTITIS	(see Bladder Infection)
DANDRUFF	Liver/Digestive Formula, change shampoos often, mucusless diet
DEAFNESS, SLIGHT	Ginkgo
DEBILITY, GEN.	Eleuthero, Adrenal/Fatigue Formula, Wild American Ginseng, Immune Deficiency Formula

DEPRESSION, MILD	St. John's wort, Energy Formula, Kava kava
DERMATITIS	Blood Purifier Formula, Echinacea Blend, Lymphatic Formula, Acne Formula, Liver/Digestive Formula
DIARRHEA	Chamomile tea, Attapulgite, Blackberry root, Black walnut
DIGESTION, POOR	Liver/Digestive Formula, Digestion/Bitters Formula 1/2 hour before meals, Relaxing Formula, Sleep Formula
DIVERTICULITIS	Digestion/Bitters Formula, Echinacea Blend, Anti-Inflammatory Formula; bowel cleansing program, wheat grass implants (see my book, *Foundations of Health,* for more information)
DIZZINESS, MILD	Ginkgo
DYSPEPSIA	Liver/Digestive Formula, Digestion/Bitters Formula
EARACHE	Echinacea Blend, Colds/Infections Formula, Mullein flower/garlic oil in ears (3 drops)
EARS, INFECTION	Echinacea Blend, Colds/Infections Formula, Mullein flower/garlic oil in ears, Usnea
ECZEMA	Liver/Digestive Formula, Milk thistle, Acne/Skin Formula
EMPHYSEMA, MILD	Respiratory Formula
ENDOMETRIOSIS	Vitex, PMS/Hormonal Formula in liquid or caplet
EXHAUSTION	Wild American ginseng, Eleuthero, Immune Deficiency Formula, Energy Formula in liquid or caplet

EYES, MILD INFECTION	Echinacea Blend, Echinacea/Vitamin C Formula, Golden seal wash externally
FERTILITY, LOW	Wild oats, Vitex, PMS/Hormonal Formula in liquid or caplet
FEVER	Echinacea Blend, Yarrow, Elder flowers, Willow bark tea
FIBROID CYSTS, BREAST, OVARIAN	Vitex, Liver Cleansing Formula, PMS/Hormonal Formula
FLATULENCE	Liver/Digestive Formula, Ginger tea, Nausea Formula
FLU	Echinacea Blend, Immune Deficiency Formula, Colds/Infections Formula, Echinacea/Vitamin C Formula
FUNGAL INFECTIONS	Echinacea Blend, Blood Purifier Formula, Usnea, Black walnut topically, internally; Tea tree oil externally
GALLSTONES, MILD	Liver/Digestive Formula, fasting
GAS, INTESTINAL AND/OR ABDOMINAL BLOATING	Liver/Digestive Formula, Ginger tea, Nausea Formula
GIARDIA	Black walnut, Echinacea Blend
GUM PROBLEMS	Mouth Formula applied to gums with soft brush before bed, rinse often with drops in water, Propolis
HAY FEVER	Hay Fever/Allergies Formula, Echinacea Blend, Blood Purifier Formula, Lymphatic Formula, Liver/Digestive Formula
HEADACHE, ACUTE	Headache Formula, Relaxing Formula

HEADACHE, CHRONIC	Headache Formula, Relaxing Formula, Sleep Formula, Relaxation techniques
HEART	Hawthorn, Heart Tonic Formula
HEMORRHOIDS	Stone root, Witch hazel (not in rubbing alcohol) externally, Horse chestnut preparation
HEPATITIS	Liver/Digestive Formula, Milk thistle (best to work with a physician and a qualified natural health practitioner)
HERPES	Echinacea Blend, Calendula, Immune Deficiency Formula, Colds/Infections Formula
HICCOUGH	Relaxing Formula, Sleep Formula, Liver/Digestive Formula
HORMONAL IMBALANCE	Vitex, PMS/Hormonal Formula in liquid or caplet, Eleuthero
HYPERACTIVITY	Relaxing Formula, Sleep Formula, Liver/Digestive Formula, Adrenal/Stress Formula
HYPERTENSION	Heart/Circulatory Formula, Relaxing Formula, Sleep Formula
HYPOCHONDRIA	Relaxing Formula, Sleep Formula, Liver/Digestive Formula, Adrenal/Stress Formula
HYPOGLYCEMIA	Eleuthero, Adrenal/Stress Formula, Adrenal/Fatigue Formula
HYSTERIA	Relaxing Formula, Sleep Formula, Valerian
IMMUNE, EXCESS	Immune Deficiency Formula

IMMUNE, DEFICIENT	Immune Deficiency Formula, Wild ginseng, Colds/Flu Formula (short term), Eleuthero, Adrenal/Fatigue Formula
IMPETIGO	Echinacea Blend, Colds/Infections Formula, Immune Deficiency Formula, more acid-forming foods in diet, Usnea
IMPOTENCE	Male toning system (Saw palmetto, Wild oats, etc.)
INDIGESTION	Liver/Digestive Formula, Digestion/Bitters Formula
INFANTS, COLIC	Chamomile tea, Catnip tea
INFECTIONS	Echinacea Blend, Colds/Infections Formula, Immune Deficiency Formula (chronic)
IRRITABLE BOWEL SYNDROME	Relaxing Formula, Sleep Formula, Valerian, Anti-Inflammatory Formula, Liver Cleansing Formula
INSECT BITES	Echinacea Blend externally, Colds/Infections Formula
INSOMNIA	Relaxing Formula, Sleep Formula, Immune Deficiency Formula, Valerian, Gotu kola
JAUNDICE	Milk thistle, Liver/Digestive Formula
JAW, TENSE	Relaxing Formula, Sleep Formula, massage, yawning
KIDNEY INFECTION OR NEPHRITIS	Adrenal/Fatigue Formula, (Bladder/Kidney Formula, light infection), Echinacea Blend, Colds/Infections Formula (best to work with a physician and qualified natural health practitioner)

LACTATION	Vitex
LARYNGITIS	Echinacea Blend, Sage tea
LEUKORRHEA	Vinegar douche, Echinacea Blend, Black walnut, Pau d'arco
LIVER, COOLING	Gentian, Digestion/Bitters Formula, Liver/Digestion Formula
LUNGS, WEAK	Respiratory Formula, Immune Deficiency Formula
LUNGS, CONGESTED	Respiratory Formula
LUPUS, MILD	Immune Deficiency Formula
MENSTRUATION, EXCESSIVE	Vitex, PMS/Hormonal Formula in liquid or caplet
MENSTRUATION, DEFICIENT (AMENORRHEA)	Vitex, PMS/Hormonal Formula in liquid or caplet
MENSTRUAL CRAMPS (DYSMENORRHEA)	Vitex, PMS/Hormonal Formula in liquid or caplet, Relaxing Formula, Sleep Formula, Valerian, Nausea Formula
MIGRAINE HEADACHE	Headache Formula, Feverfew, Relaxing Formula, Sleep Formula, Liver/Digestive Formula
METABOLISM, BALANCE	Adrenal/Fatigue Formula, Cayenne caplets (if too slow)
MORNING SICKNESS	Chinese rhubarb (small amount), Nausea Formula
MOUTH, SORES	Mouth Care Formula, Propolis, Echinacea Blend

MUCUS, EXCESS	Respiratory Formula
MUSCLES, TIGHT, SORE	Relaxing Formula, Sleep Formula, Valerian, California poppy
NAUSEA, GENERAL	Nausea Formula, Golden seal (not during pregnancy)
NERVOUS SYSTEM EXHAUSTION	Relaxing Formula, Sleep Formula, Wild oats, Adrenal/Fatigue Formula
NERVOUS SYSTEM TONIFY	Relaxing Formula, Sleep Formula, Valerian, Adrenal/Fatigue Formula, sea vegetables
NERVOUS SYSTEM, TOO STIMULATED	Relaxing Formula, Sleep Formula
NEURALGIA	Relaxing Formula, Sleep Formula, Castor oil packs, hot/cold applications, Valerian, analgesic oils externally
NEURITIS	Analgesic oils (Chamomile) externally, Relaxing Formula, Sleep Formula, St. John's wort
NIGHTMARES	Passion flower, Relaxing Formula, Sleep Formula, Liver/Digestive Formula
NOSE, PLUGGED	Respiratory Formula, Echinacea Blend, Colds/Infections Formula
NUMBNESS	Ginger compresses, Wild American ginseng
ODOR, BREATH	Mouth Care Formula, Digestion/Bitters Formula, Laxative/Bowel Tonic (if constipated), Liver/Digestive Formula
OVARIAN CYST	Vitex, PMS/Hormonal Formula in liquid or caplet

OVERWEIGHT	Liver/Digestive Formula, Eleuthero, Adrenal/Fatigue Formula, Cayenne caplets, reduce calories, Bladderwrack
PAIN, RELIEVE	Willow bark extract, Valerian, Roman chamomile oil externally, tincture internally
PALPITATIONS	Heart Tonic Formula, Hawthorn
PNEUMONIA	Echinacea Blend, Echinacea/Vitamin C Formula, Colds/Infections Formula, Immune Deficiency Formula, Usnea
POISONING	Echinacea Blend, Colds/Infections Formula (full course), Immune Deficiency Formula, cleansing, sweating, colonics
PROSTATE IMBALANCE	Bladder/Kidney Formula, Echinacea Blend
PROTECTIVES	Echinacea Blend, Colds/Infections Formula, Immune Deficiency Formula, Eleuthero, Adrenal/Fatigue Formula
PSORIASIS	Milk thistle, Liver/Digestive Formula, Acne/Skin Formula
PSYCHIATRIC	Ginkgo, St. John's wort, Kava kava
PYORRHEA	Mouth Care Formula, Echinacea Blend, Propolis
REJUVENATION	Wild ginseng, Adrenal/Fatigue Formula, Ten Ginsengs Formula
RHEUMATISM	Feverfew, hydrotherapy, diet
SCABIES	10 % sulfur ointment for 3 nights, Colds/Infections Formula
SCALP	Milk thistle, Liver/Digestive Formula, change shampoo often, hydrotherapy

SCIATICA	Hydrotherapy, Relaxing Formula, Sleep Formula, Valerian, essential oils—clary sage or chamomile (a few drops added to St. John's wort oil) externally
SEASICKNESS	Nausea/Motion Sickness Formula
SEDATIVES	Relaxing Formula, Sleep Formula, Valerian
SEXUAL ENERGY, TO DECREASE	Skullcap
SEXUAL ENERGY, TO INCREASE	Damiana, Energy Formula, Aphrodisiac Formula
SHINGLES	Echinacea Blend, Colds/Infections Formula, Immune Deficiency Formula, St. John's wort
SKIN, ACNE	Hydrotherapy, no soap on affected areas, Colds/Infections Formula, Immune Deficiency Formula, Adrenal/Fatigue, Vitex, Blood Purifier Formula, Acne/Skin Formula
SKIN, RASHES	Calendula cream
SKIN, SOOTHE	Chamomile, Calendula creams
SLEEPING AIDS	Relaxing Formula, Sleep Formula, Valerian
SPASMS	Relaxing Formula, Sleep Formula, hydrotherapy
SPLEEN, TONIC	Echinacea Blend, Red root (*Ceanothus americanus*)
STIMULANTS	Energy Formula, Cayenne
STINGS	Calendula cream, Plantain or Comfrey poultice

STOMACH, ULCERS	Chamomile tea, Licorice tea, Marshmallow root
STRESS	Adrenal/Stress Formula, Relaxing Formula, Valerian
STYE	Echinacea Blend, Colds/Infections Formula
STYPTICS	Yarrow leaf powder, Cayenne
TEETHING	Calendula, Chamomile
TENDONS	Hydrotherapy, Horsetail extract, Nettles
THROAT, SORE	Sage/lemon peel/ honey tea, Echinacea Blend, Colds/Infections Formula, Echinacea/Vitamin C Formula
THYROID, HYPER	Bladderwrack, sea vegetables, Eleuthero
THYROID, HYPO	Bladderwrack, sea vegetables, Guggulu
TINNITIS	Ginkgo
TONIC, GENERAL	Eleuthero, Immune Deficiency Formula, Adrenal/Fatigue Formula, Adrenal/Stress Formula
TONSILS, INFECTED	Echinacea Blend, Colds/Infections Formula, Usnea
TOOTHACHE	Clove oil, Plantain and clay poultice, Echinacea Blend
TRANQUILIZERS, MILD	Relaxing Formula, Sleep Formula, Valerian
TRICHAMONAS	Black walnut, Colds/Infections Formula, Echinacea (concentrated)

URINARY INFECTION	Bladder/Kidney Formula, Colds/Infections Formula, Echinacea Blend, Echinacea/Vitamin C Formula
UTERINE CYSTS (FIBROIDS)	Vitex, PMS/Hormonal Formula in liquid or caplet
VAGINA, DRY	Vitex, PMS/Hormonal Formula in liquid or caplet
VAGINA, DISCHARGE	Vinegar douche, Usnea, PMS/Hormonal Formula in liquid or caplet, Echinacea Blend, Colds/Infections Formula
VERTIGO	Ginkgo
VIRAL INFECTION	Colds/Infections Formula, Echinacea Blend, Golden seal, Echinacea/Vitamin C Formula, Anti-Viral Formula
VITALITY, LOW	Wild ginseng, Adrenal/Fatigue Formula, Immune Deficiency Formula, Ten Ginsengs Formula
WARTS	Echinacea Blend, Colds/Infections Formula
WOUNDS	Usnea, Echinacea Blend, Gotu kola
YEAST INFECTION	Vitex, PMS/Hormonal Formula in liquid or caplet, vinegar douche

REFERENCES

1.   Hobbs, C.R. 1990. *Usnea: The Herbal Antibiotic!*. Capitola, CA: Botanica Press.

2.   Parke, Davis & Company. 1924. *Manual of Therapy* (3rd ed.).
     Detroit: Parke, Davis & Co.

3.   Carbin, C.E., et al. 1990. Treatment of benign prostatic hyperplasia
     with phytosterols. *Br. J. Urol.* 66:639-41.

4.   Papas, P.N., et al. 1966. *Southwest. Med.* 47: 17.

5.   Hobbs, C. 1989. *Echinacea Handbook*. Capitola, CA: Botanica Press.

6.   Bye, R.A., Jr. & E. Linares. 1986. Ethnobotanical notes from the valley of San Luis,
     Colorado. *J. Ethnobiol* 6: 289-306.

7.   Timbrook, J. 1987. Virtuous herbs: plants in Chumash medicine.
     J. Ethnobiol. 7: 171-80.

8.   Mead, G.R. 1972. *The ethnobotany of the California Indians*. University of
     Northern Colorado, Occasional Publications in Anthropology, Ethnology Series 30: 18.

9.   Moerman, D.E. 1986. *Medicinal Plants of Native America*, 2 vols.
     University of Michigan Museum of Anthropology Technical Reports 19: 228.

10. Hobbs, *Echinacea Handbook*, op. cit.

11. Tierra, M. 1988. *Planetary Herbology*. Santa Fe: Lotus Press.

12. Merck & Co. 1907. *Merck's 1907 Index*. Rahway, NJ: Merck & Co.

13. Hobbs, C. 1988. *Natural Liver Therapy*. Capitola, CA: Botanica Press.

14. Hammerl H., O. Pichler and M. Studlar. 1971.
     "Report on the action of silymarin in liver diseases." *Med. Klin.* 66: 1204-8.

15. Magliulo, E., B. Gagliardi and G.P. Fiori. 1978. "Results of a double blind study on the
     effect of silymarin in the treatment of acute viral hepatitis." *Med. Klin.* 73: 1060-5.

16. Poser, Von Gunther. 1971. "Experience in the treatment of chronic hepatopathies
     with silymarin." *Arzneim.-Forsch.* 21: 1209-12.

17. Massacci, P. 1967. Corriere Farm 22: 69; through Chem. Abstr. 67:89667b.

18. Hammerl, W.H., et al. 1973. *Wien. Med. Wochenschr.* 123: 601.

19. Schwabe, W. 1959. *Arzneimittel-Forsch* 9: 376.

20. Madaus, G. 1938. *Lehrbuch der biologischen Heilmittel*.
     Reprinted by Georg Olms Verlag, NY (1976), pp. 2678-80.

21. Perry, L.M. 1980. *Medicinal Plants of East and Southeast Asia.*
Cambridge: The MIT Press.

22. Chadha, Y.R., chief ed. 1952-88. *The Wealth of India* (Raw Materials), 11 vols.
New Delhi: Publications and Information Directorate, CSIR.

23. Wren, R.C. 1988. *Potter's New Cyclopaedia of Botanical Drugs and Preparations.*
Wigan, England: Potter's Ltd.

24. Vogel, G. 1981. "A peculiarity among the flavonoids—silymarin, a compound active on
the liver." *Proceedings of the International Bioflavonoid Symposium.* Munich, p. 472.

25. Theiss, P. & B. Theiss. 1989. *The Family Herbal.* Rochester, VT: Healing Arts Press.

26. For a complete review, see: Hobbs, *The Echinacea Handbook,* op. cit.

27. Available through Botanica Press, Box 742, Capitola, CA 95010.

28. Leung, A. 1980. *Encyclopedia of Common Natural Ingredients.*
New York, NY: John Wiley & Sons.

29. James, R. 1747. *Pharmacopoeia Universalis.* London: J. Hodges, at the
Looking-Glass.

30. Brunton, T.L. 1893. *A Text-book of Pharmacology,*
Therapeutics and Materia Medica. London: Macmillan and Co., p. 1019.

31. Dash, V.B. 1980. *Materia Medica of Ayurveda.*
New Delhi: Concept Publishing Co., p. 608.

32. Ellingwood, F. 1898. *American Materia Medica, Therapeutics and Pharmacognosy.*
Reprinted by Portland, OR: Eclectic Medical Publications, 1983.

33. Felter & Lloyd, op. cit.

34. Leung, op. cit.

35. ibid.

36. Goodman, L.S. & A. Gilman. 1966. *The Pharmacological Basis of Therapeutics.*
New York: The Macmillan Co., p. 354-66.

37. Leung, op. cit.

38. Weiss, R.F. 1988. *Herbal Medicine.* Beaconsfield, England: Beaconsfield Publishers Ltd.

39. ibid.

40. Chang, H.-M. & P. But. 1986. *Pharmacology and Applications of Chinese Materia*
Medica. Philadelphia: World Scientific.

41. Mittman, P. 1990. Randomized, double-blind study of freeze-dried *Urtica dioica*
in the treatment of allergic rhinitis. *Planta Med.* 56: 44-7.

42. Chang & But, op. cit.

43. Hobbs, golden seal, op. cit.

44. Chang & But, op. cit.

45. Hobbs, C. 1988. *Medicinal Mushrooms.* Capitola, CA: Botanica Press.

46. Bo, Li & B. Yun-sun. 1980. *Fungi Pharmacopoeia* (Sinica). Oakland, CA: The Kinoko Co.

47. Chang & But, op. cit.

48. Sun, Y., et al. 1983. Immune restoration and/or augmentation of local graft versus host reaction by Traditional Chinese medicinal herbs. *Cancer* 52: 70-3.

49. Look for books by Louise Hay, Bernie Siegel and the Journal, *Advances.*

50. Locke, S. & D. Colligan. 1986. *The Healer Within.* New York: A Mentor Book.

51. Any books by Paul C. Bragg, such as *The Miracle of Fasting.*

52. *Lawrence Review of Natural Products,* Nov. 1986.

53. Harnaj, E. V. New Apitherapy Research, 2nd International Symposium on Apitherapy, Bucharest, Sept. 2-7th, 1976. Bucharest: Apimondia Pub. House.

54. Hobbs, C. 1990. *Usnea—the Herbal Antibiotic.* Capitola, CA: Botanica Press.

55. Chadha, Y.R., chief ed. 1952-88. *The Wealth of India* (Raw Materials), 11 vols. New Delhi: Publications and Information Directorate, CSIR.

56. Hobbs, C. 1990. *Vitex—The Women's Herb.* Capitola, CA: Botanica Press.

57. Felter & Lloyd, op. cit.

58. Grontved, A., et al. 1900. "Ginger root against seasickness." *Acta oto-laryngol.* 105: 45-49.

59. Mowrey, D.B. & D.E. Clayson. 1982. *Lancet* ii: 655.

60. Lust, J. 1974. *The Herb Book.* NY: Bantam Books.

61. Moore, M. 1982. *Herbal Repertory in Clinical Practice.* Santa Fe: Institute of Traditional Medicine.

62. Hobbs, C. 1989. Valerian—A Literature Review. *HerbalGram* 21: 19-35.

63. List, P.H. and L. Hörhammer. 1973. *Hagers Handbuch der Pharmazeutischen Praxis,* 7 vols. New York: Springer-Verlag.

64. List & Hörhammer, op. cit.

65. Hobbs, C. 1990. Getting to the Heart of Hawthorn. *HerbalGram* 22: 19-33.

66. Gathercoal, E.N. & H.W. Youngken. 1942. Check list of native and introduced drug plants in the U.S. Chicago: National Research Council.

67. Felter, H.W. & J.U. Lloyd. 1898. *King's American Dispensatory.* Cincinnati: The Ohio Valley Co.

68. Leung, op. cit.

69. Chang & But, op. cit.

70. Hobbs, C. 1990. Golden seal in early American medical botany. *Pharmacy in History* 32: 79-82.

71. Smith, F.P. & G.A. Stuart. 1973. *Chinese Medicinal Herbs.* San Francisco: Georgetown Press.

72. Chang & But, op. cit.

73. Bensky, D. & A. Gamble. 1986. *Chinese Herbal Medicine Materia Medica.* Seattle: Eastland Press.

74. Felter, op. cit.

75. Personal observation of the author.

76. Brekhman, I.I. 1980. *Man and biologically active substances.* New York: Pergamon Press.

77. Farnsworth, N., et al. 1985. "Siberian ginseng (*Eleutherococcus senticosus*): current status as an adaptogen." In: *Economic and Medicinal Plant Research,* vol. 1. Orlando: Academic Press, Inc.

78. Bensky, op. cit.

79. Chang & But, op. cit.

80. Hobbs, C. 1986. *Milk Thistle—The Liver Herb.* Capitola, CA: Botanica Press.

81. Weiss, op. cit.

82. Santana, C.F. et al. 1968. Antitumoral and toxicological properties of extracts of bark and various wood components of Pau d'arco (*Tabebuia vellanedae*). *Rev Inst Antibiot* 8:89-94.

83. Harnaj, op. cit.

84. Farnsworth, op. cit.

85. Hobbs, Valerian, op. cit.